UNDERSTANDING ANOREXIA NERVOS

Peter Dally is an eminent psychiatrist and Britain's leading expert on the treatment of anorexia nervosa.

Joan Gomez is a consultant psychiatrist in private practice in London.

Related titles published by Faber

SURVIVING ADOLESCENCE
A Handbook for Adolescents and Their Parents
by Peter Bruggen and Charles O'Brien

SECRETS IN THE FAMILY
by Lily Pincus and Christopher Dare

HELPING FAMILIES
by Peter Bruggen and Charles O'Brien

ANOREXIA NERVOSA: The Broken Circle
by Ann Erichsen

DRUG USE AND ABUSE
by James Willis

DEPRESSION
by Robert Romanis

AGORAPHOBIA
by Ruth Hurst Vose

MULTIPLE SCLEROSIS
Exploring Sickness and Health
by Elizabeth Forsythe

EVERYWOMAN
A Gynaecological Guide for Life
by Derek Llewellyn-Jones

PREPARING FOR PREGNANCY
by Philip J. Robarts

YOUR CHILD'S HEALTH
by Ivan Blumenthal

FOOD FACTS AND FIGURES
A Comprehensive Guide to Healthy Eating
by Jill Davis and J. W. T. Dickerson

Understanding
Anorexia Nervosa and Obesity

A sense of proportion

Peter Dally
MB, FRCP, FRCPsych., DPM

Joan Gomez
MB, FRCPsych., DPM

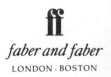

faber and faber
LONDON · BOSTON

First published in 1990
by Faber and Faber Limited
3 Queen Square London WC1N 3AU

Photoset by Parker Typesetting Service Leicester
Printed in Great Britain by
Richard Clay Ltd Bungay Suffolk

Peter Dally and Joan Gomez are hereby identified as authors of this work in
accordance with Section 77 of the Copyright, Designs and Patents Act 1988.

A CIP record for this book is available from the British Library

ISBN 0–571–15473–5

Contents

Preface

The more affluent the country, the greater and more widespread the concern of its women – and some men – over their weight, the shape of their bodies, and what they consume. Weight is never far from the thoughts of most women today. One declares she is overweight, yet eating nothing, another that her thighs are enormous despite the hours she devotes to massage and esoteric exercises. Many of these complaints seem unjustified to an observer, but to the complainer they are very real. New diets and treatments are constantly devised and sought. The media never cease to proclaim that every woman can retain her youth and attraction by preserving her weight and figure.

On the other side of the coin is the individual whose fears lead her to diet to excess, even to death; anorexia nervosa is rife among intelligent young women today. However thin they become they rarely complain; it is their worried relatives who object and drag them into the limelight. Linked to this strange disorder is bulimia nervosa, seemingly a new disease but in fact an ancient one, politely kept in family cupboards until now.

Why are eating disorders so common? Why are women more prone to them than men? The causes are multiple and complex. New theories purporting to explain all come and go. Feminists believe the problems to be illusory, created by women, sheeplike, giving undue importance to men's expectations of women; that a woman must be thin to attract and be successful. This certainly plays a part in eating disorders, but a small one. So too with the theme of childhood sexual abuse which, enthusiasts maintain, explains everything. Not a few women with anorexia nervosa/ bulimia or obesity admit to incidents in childhood which amount to sexual abuse; how much is real or elaborated from fantasy, remains as much a problem to us as it did to Freud. And even when sexual abuse is accepted as a *fait accompli*, its role in the eating disorder remains conjectural, a part only of the causal jigsaw puzzle.

In the chapters ahead we attempt to illuminate the field of eating disorders, to make sense of the different aberrations of appetite and eating behaviour, and discuss forms of treatment and help.

Part One
Anorexia Nervosa

Chapter 1

Introduction:
What Anorexia Nervosa is

We eat for many reasons. The most obvious is hunger. Hunger, that gut sensation that can range from pleasurable to frankly painful, builds up slowly in the absence of food and becomes ever stronger until satisfied. It is a complex of physical sensations; stirring of the stomach and intestines, progressing to general irritability and restlessness, combined with cold and fatigue. Some people develop headache, others feel nauseous; but know that food will put this right. Hunger can be diminished, or even abolished for a time, by absorbing activities, or by powerful emotions unconnected with food. Sooner or later it breaks through and dominates thought and activity. The more starved man is, the more readily is he satisfied by simple, unsophisticated foods. A desire for exotic dishes and sauces arises only when hunger is not extreme. As hunger is assuaged, so appetite takes increasing charge.

Appetite and habit dictate what food we fancy or reject. As remarked in 1565 by Thomas Coggan, respected physician to the Court of Elizabeth: 'Custom bringeth liking. For what the stomach liketh it greedily desireth; and having received it, encloseth it about until it be duly concocted. Which thing is the cause that meat and drink wherein we have great delighte, though it be much worse than other, yet it doth us more good.'

Appetite anticipates pleasure – from the meal or from the next mouthful. While appetite continues, so will eating, even if sufficient nutriment has already been consumed. Thus while appetite and hunger are intimately related, on occasion one may totally dominate eating behaviour. A starving man will usually eat anything he can lay his hands on, however repellent the food may seem to him under normal circumstances; for instance, cannibalism among survivors, or horse-dung casserole in the siege of Leningrad. It is normal enough to continue eating a little longer, after hunger has been fully met, to satisfy appetite. However, some people may continue to eat remorselessly and compulsively, guzzling everything in sight until the belly feels at bursting point. So strong may be the compulsion to go on eating that such people may make themselves vomit to provide gastric space.

Occasionally, appetite may conflict with hunger in an inhibitory way, making food repulsive: the situation of the traveller in the desert, offered a stew of fat, white maggots, or the proverbial sheep's eye. Sometimes a person may starve in the midst of plenty, as happens in anorexia nervosa. Appetite and hunger combined tempt the sufferer to eat, but not strongly enough to crush her fear of the consequences.

Appetite is a more complex mental force than hunger. Hunger develops when physiological changes in the body signal that more fuel is needed. Animals in the wild maintain their weights at a constant level because hunger, not appetite, is the controlling force in them. Only domestic pets and other captives become fat. Appetite is not basically concerned with energy balance as hunger is. It arises from habit and past experiences with food. Cream cakes, say, through association with pleasurable and happy childhood treats, may be compulsively craved by the adult when he is unhappy or lonely and longs to regress.

Appetite links food with memories and fantasies; with magic and superstition; with love, power and prestige; with happiness and also with misery. More precisely, appetite is influenced by emotions and needs unconnected, or only tenuously so, with nutritional requirements. Coleridge summed up one side of the matter when he declared that a man 'cannot have a good conscience who refuses apple dumplings'. Doctor Johnson, with his accustomed complacency, said: 'Some people have a foolish way of not minding, or pretending not to mind, what they eat. For my part, I mind my belly very studiously, and very carefully, for I look upon it, that he who does not mind his belly will hardly mind anything else.' He also suggested that one should leave the table while still feeling the capacity to consume a Bath bun. But habit, good sense and the state of the belly are by no means the most important aspects of appetite; appetite dies if even the most delicious food is offered by someone with whom you are at odds. In anorexia nervosa, the conflict between parents and child turns off appetite at the family table, although hunger is allowed some sway in private.

Severe hunger, particularly if it is sustained, narrows actions and thoughts. Most people today strike a reasonable balance between their appetite and hunger, although at any time appetite is apt to run amok when strong, unsatisfied emotional demands seek an outlet through eating. Food is then apt to become the centre of the person's life, dominating thoughts and actions in an apparently irrational way, while it provides a means of partial satisfaction to other, less readily fulfilled, emotional needs.

The agony and struggle of the compulsive eater resisting the lure of a packet of biscuits (particularly if it has already been opened); a midnight feast of bread and jam; Cornflakes and sugar and milk; chocolate to bite and then melt in the mouth – all are ultimately in vain. The real enemy is not food, but lies elsewhere.

Starving people eat silently, not only because their mouths are full but because nothing else for the moment can penetrate their senses. Only when hunger begins to fall can such people relax sufficiently to begin to communicate.

Most of us are not starving, however hungry we may be. When we eat we like to do so with other people; with those we love, are fond of and trust; with those we want to get to know better or to do business with. Sharing an enjoyable experience is a basis for communication. Many people can't be bothered to cook or eat a balanced nutritional meal when they are by themselves, which is one of the problems met by those concerned with old or sick people who live alone. But some people, particularly women, when they are on their own, even if only for part of the day, become bored and vaguely dissatisfied and are faced with the opposite problem. Like St Anthony in the desert, they are constantly tempted – but by food, not bodies. Food is, of course, more available. They nibble, have repeated snacks of tea and biscuits or cake, or suddenly 'go mad' and stuff themselves with anything they can find in the fridge or larder, salad foods coming low in the list.

'I don't know when to stop' is their common complaint. These unfortunate people feel as though they have two sets of stop/go eating signals inside them – one set that operates correctly in the presence of other people, and one that goes haywire when they are on their own. In fact, they rely upon what other people do to regulate their own behaviour and are lost without a 'reference man'. Since they cannot have someone else at hand 24 hours a day, inevitably many of them become fat. Such sufferers are not able to endure their own company for any length of time. They begin to feel restless, bored, anxious (feelings reminiscent of hunger). It is difficult for them to relax or to settle down with a book or become absorbed in work unconnected with food. Eating relieves their discomfort, and temporarily subdues tension and boredom, but the more this happens, the more likely it is to occur in the future; and the more difficult it becomes to stop.

Most meals are sociable occasions; not only is food shared, but news, ideas, plans and feelings. Those who are much alone, because of infirmity or widowhood, usually take a tray by the television set, or to the fireside 'for companionship'. For someone to eat alone habitually, from choice, is unusual; a sign that all is not well. It indicates that he has excluded himself from his social group – or been rejected. Lonely children always eat their sweets alone, reluctant to share; compulsive eaters stuff in shameful secret; girls with anorexia nervosa prefer to eat their tiny morsels alone, away from the rest of the family. It is a sure sign of family discord when mother and father eat their meals at different times or apart. It is difficult to eat and enjoy a meal with someone you dislike or resent.

We share our food and communicate during mealtimes from the moment we are born. It is impossible not to do so, since the child is totally dependent on his mother, or mother surrogate, for the preparation and delivery of his food for many years. The way a child is fed and the ease and enjoyment with which he accepts his food probably reflects the relationship that exists between him and his mother. Later on it involves whoever else is present at the meal. In turn, the child's behaviour at mealtimes, whether his attitude is mainly one of acceptance or rejection, must influence how others feel towards him. It is difficult for a mother not to become angry and anxious when her child screams or vomits at every meal, however fond and protective of him she is at heart. Mealtimes are frequently something of a battleground, and the giving and taking of food shift from the purely biological to the symbolic expression of emotional needs, demands and conflicts. The unhappy, anxious child may convey his distress by refusing to eat, by throwing back food into his mother's face. Conversely, he may guzzle insatiably and long, never achieving the satisfaction he seeks, and probably becoming fat. The happy child does not, of course, always feed as perfectly as his mother would wish, but there is, by and large, a mutual pleasure in meals, contentment and relaxation that communicates itself to all those present.

Meals are an important part of family life. They reflect and reinforce emotional security and solidarity. Through the presence of guests, they help a child move gradually from his family into a wider social world. The ritual of mealtimes emphasizes the role and status of those present. Children respond to the knowledge that they are now considered responsible and 'grown up' enough to eat with their elders. They recognize that they must now behave in an acceptable manner and consider the needs and feelings of those present at the meal table, otherwise they are liable to be excluded – at any rate when their parents are entertaining.

Where people sit at the table, who carves the joint, who is served first or last – these are important aspects that help to formalize mealtimes yet keep them familiar and easy. The mechanics of dinner must be smoothly running for conversation to become an integral part of it. Indeed, when the host or hostess loses control, whether it be at a children's party or a turbulent adult dinner, chaos is likely to develop. Communication, except of the most primitive kind, comes to a close and is replaced by childlike patterns of behaviour. Food is then neglected.

Some people find it difficult to eat normally outside a formal framework. They require the familiar structure and accustomed cues to know when to eat and when to stop. Put them at a picnic or let them eat alone and they are lost. The traditional Englishman, dressing for dinner in the desert, is perhaps attempting to recapture his bearings as are those people who take a folding table and chairs and eat, sitting bolt upright, in a car park near a beauty spot. The picnic hamper with plates and knives and forks is a compromise.

A meal may proclaim the prosperity and values of the host. A slap-up meal is organized with enormous effort to impress an important business acquaintance or he is taken to an expensive restaurant where not only his host's wealth but his discriminating tastes are displayed. Food in this instance indicates not only friendship and trust, but also generosity and power. It is this combination that some fat people, notably plump businessmen, find so particularly difficult to resist. A 'bay window' stomach with a heavy gold watch-chain draped across it was the *sine qua non* of prosperity at the beginning of this century.

Sometimes children compete among themselves to see who can eat the most, to assert their greater capacity and therefore superiority. This is analogous with the boasting about beer consumption among young men. A child who eats enormously is likely to attract parental attention and semi-admiration; his mother cannot help but be secretly somewhat gratified at first. Huge quantities of food may be consumed, however, and the compulsion to eat in quantity may grow stronger unless a perceptive parent intervenes. Children who gorge habitually are always emotionally insecure and the maladaptive response of eating much more food than they need when they are unsure of themselves or upset frequently persists into adult life.

Parents and hostesses are pleased to see their food eaten up and their culinary efforts appreciated. It is most upsetting to a hostess for the food that she has chosen and prepared to be refused or only sampled. The implication is that she has failed to please and is herself rejected. No matter how much the guest protests that he is allergic to *boeuf Stroganoff*, has an upset stomach, is on a special diet from his doctor, or has religious scruples, his hosts are liable to feel hurt.

Special foods or dishes help to cement communities and preserve national, religious and group solidarity. For Jewish people the meal table is the centre of family unity; that the food is kosher reinforces their sense of racial and religious distinctiveness. All the major religions – Christian, Moslem and Buddhist, for instance – have special feast-days and times of fasting. Immigrants to a new land, apprehensive and uncertain of their acceptance and survival, often preserve their food habits rigidly long after they have absorbed and become familiar with the customs and values of their new country. Food habits seem to be as strong as language, if not more so, in preserving family and racial traditions and unity, and familiar foods, like familiar words, are reassuring and comforting and bring a sense of belonging among those with whom they are shared. The small colony of White Russian *emigrés* who have lived in New York since the 1920s still serve special Russian dishes (despite ingredients being hard to get) and practise their mother tongue at the family table. Pakistanis long since settled in England behave similarly.

It is always the insecure, the lowest socio-economic classes and young children who cling most tenaciously to the food they know best, and it is often extremely difficult to alter their eating habits because they fiercely resist any change. Attempts to introduce new and nutritionally better foods into deprived areas of the population require considerable skill and understanding to succeed. Trying to persuade a child to eat a new dish can be hard, especially if he is anxious or unhappy. A sudden change of food, say on a foreign holiday, is met by an upturned nose and uncomplimentary comments and asides. 'Why can't we have fish and chips instead of worms?' demanded a 5-year-old English girl in Rome, upset by new surroundings and longing for the secure world of home. For an adult, the food he ate as a child has a nostalgic appeal. One successful, self-made millionaire still hankers after bread fried in bacon fat which in his youth was all that his hard-pressed mother could afford.

Rigid childhood eating habits persist throughout life for some people, especially those with a long-standing disorder such as anorexia nervosa. Every meal is the same and any deviation from the familiar is greeted by a storm of recrimination. A mother proudly producing a soufflé for the first time may find that no one will even try it. She does not repeat the experiment. Such people's lives centre around their food, for psychological security demands familiarity and sameness. In some families, perhaps because of a bad-tempered father demanding high standards at table, mealtimes come to be associated with fear and tension. Children brought up in these circumstances are liable to react in later life to stressful situations by inability to eat or vomiting whatever they have taken in. Some cases of secondary anorexia nervosa develop in this way.

Anxiety has the effect of drying up secretions in the mouth and stomach, lessening the contractions of the stomach at the prospect of food and reducing acuity of taste and smell. How then can it be that some people 'eat their way out' of gloom and anxiety? Think of that baby, so fretful before being fed, gurgling with contentment afterwards with all its tensions gone:

> '. . . Oh, he had swooned,
> Drunken from pleasure's nipple.'

Keats's lines were written from self-observation: 'talking of pleasure, this moment I was writing with one hand, and with the other holding to my mouth a nectarine – Good God, how fine – it went down soft, pulpy, slushy, oozy – all its delicious embonpoint melted down my throat like a beautiful strawberry.' The early, blissful months of post-prandial satisfaction become organized and reorganized in the brain by association, fantasy and, as likely as not, pure chance, so that when unpleasant emotions later arise they call forth a craving for food. Keats may have lost his appetite when upset, but his description of the nectarine brings to mind the behaviour of the unhappy 14-stone woman who crams down biscuits, butter and jam in the middle of the night for 'a lovely feeling of comfort and warmth'.

Some people feel lost without something in their mouth. It helps if they chew food slowly, tasting and feeling each mouthful for as long as possible. Chewing-gum is sometimes useful, but it is of the wrong consistency and lacks the delight of swallowing. A sense of tension possesses them, especially when alone, only to be subdued by constant 'snacking' or excessive smoking.

Can we attribute such faulty eating habits to childhood deprivation? The trouble with such a theory is that all of us have had difficulties or been deprived, in one way or another, at some time. We simply do not know why some children react one way and some another, to the ups and downs and inevitable tensions of family life. It is fashionable but usually unhelpful to blame the mother. The mental processes concerned in the development of an individual's instinctive behaviour are many and complex and still not fully understood; all one can say with certainty in this area is that once the links between food and emotion have been forged, a pattern of eating behaviour has become established. Repetition of that behaviour fixes it ever more strongly in the nervous system.

Much of our eating depends on habit and routine quite apart from whether we feel hungry. We eat either because everyone else is doing so, or a meal has been prepared at home, or because we are due for a break at work. A bell or gong signalling that it is lunchtime, the sight and smell of food, talk of food, or reading a recipe in a magazine – all these may turn our thoughts towards eating. How many of us can pass a baker's shop smelling of bread still hot from the oven without wanting at least a bite? And there must be few children who can resist the lure of a confectioner's window, spangled with shiny chocolate beans, crumbling chunks of fudge, jelly babies and multi-coloured Liquorice Allsorts. We are surrounded by food and temptations to eat. Sixty per cent of television commercials show happy, beautiful people eating or offering goodies to their children or their partners.

We are certainly nudged from within by our internal signals, but in today's affluent society we are bombarded constantly by external inducements to eat.

Chapter 2

Causes of Anorexia Nervosa

Anorexia nervosa has a number of causes. Psychological difficulties can arise in three separate areas: (1) the individual's psychosomatic nature; (2) the structure of her family relationships; and (3) cultural values, especially those proclaimed through the popular media. When two or more coincide the cumulative effect may overwhelm the individual who then regresses to an earlier, more immature stage of her life, and her behaviour and thinking become more childlike.

Psychosomatic influences

There is considerable variation in the age at which people mature and reach puberty; today most girls start to menstruate between 11 and 15, considerably earlier than in Victorian and Edwardian times. In 95 per cent of cases anorexia nervosa develops at or after puberty. The condition can begin just before puberty, when hormonal changes have already begun to remould their bodies, but before signs of menstruation. Stresses within the family are likely to be particularly strong in such cases.

Puberty and adolescence are naturally stressful for most teenagers; there are psychological and social pressures requiring readjustment and changes in lifestyle. As the child becomes adult she, or he, struggles to assert herself and develop a firm identity, and gain control of her inner and outer worlds, so often at variance with one another.

The adolescent who cannot cope retreats into herself and withdraws from the outside world. The one who goes on to develop anorexia nervosa organizes her life around her body. A conviction grows that if she can control her weight she will control her life. To be thin – she sees, reads and hears – is desirable, a necessary precondition for success. She therefore relentlessly pursues the goal of thinness and in the process drops the 'burdens of womanhood' (Sheila MacLeod), and gains the admiration of friends; to some parts of society the anorexic has taken on the role of romantic heroine. At first she has a sense of liberation. But alas this does not last and sooner or later she finds herself imprisoned and restrained by insurmountable mental barriers.

Because areas in the hypothalamus are known to influence eating behaviour and the onset of puberty and menstruation, it is tempting to postulate an organic basis to anorexia nervosa, some as yet undiscovered disorder in the hypothalamus. It is most unlikely to exist. Hypothalamic functions are undoubtedly disturbed in anorexia nervosa, but this is due not only to primary psychological influences but the weight loss itself.

Her family

The family of anyone with a neurotic or psychosomatic disorder must accept some responsibility for the condition. It is they, after all, who have largely shaped and fashioned their child's personality, and given rise to her expectations and ambitions. Every family behaves characteristically within its own circle, and its members relate to one another stereotypically.

Anorexic families, containing one or more cases of anorexia nervosa, often have a typical pattern. Family members are emotionally over-involved with one another, known as 'enmeshment', so that the anorexic feels swamped and unable to express her individuality in any reasonable way. The family structure is a rigid one, and the parents seem reluctant to alter their attitudes to their children as they grow up. They protect them too much, the overprotection even extending to their food. They constantly harp on nutrition and what should and should not be eaten. Often one finds that a close relative has had anorexia nervosa or is notorious in the family for his or her bizarre food fads and eccentricities, is a martyr to so-called food allergies, or devotes his or her culinary energies to following the latest dietary fashion and eating only fat-free foods grown by natural means. Mealtime conversations often centre around food and weight.

Open family conflict is not tolerated and tensions and disagreements are quickly brushed under the carpet. Family pressures thus prevent the potential anorexic from asserting herself openly and squash every attempt at expressing herself as an individual. She is forced into passive resistance, into taking on the whole family at its most vulnerable point, the meal table. By refusing to eat she signifies her resentment and frustration and the family is made to acknowledge that there is a problem. At the same time the anorexic steadfastly maintains in the family tradition that she is fine and not in the least put out or worried, and there is no justification for the family's concern. The effect on the family can be like a volcano erupting with burning lava sliding ever further afield. The anorexic's behaviour starkly reveals the tensions and conflicts within the family. Sometimes this is more than the family can tolerate and it is destroyed as a functioning unit; occasionally rigidity and enmeshment increase and other members of the family develop psychosomatic illness or become overtly depressed and suicidal; more often anorexia nervosa loosens the restricting chains enmeshing the family and allows it a new freedom and chance to grow.

Socio-cultural influences

These are probably largely responsible for anorexia nervosa being predominantly a female disease. Modern young women, successful in life and admired by their peers, are portrayed as slim and elegant; to be overweight is a sure sign of failure. A careful diet is a *sine qua non* for health, wealth and happiness.

Until puberty, the child is encouraged to keep up her strength and health by frequent snacks and regular meals. Once she reaches adolescence all this changes and her weight and slimming become serious preoccupations. She weighs herself, looks at herself and slides between success and failure, envies the slim figures of her friends and feels both relief and anxiety at the sight of an overweight companion. Then, suddenly, with new-found determination she resolves to become *thin*, seriously begins to diet; her weight falls away, and she proudly reveals herself – *en route* she is sure to perfect thinness. On all sides society encourages her; the models have smaller and smaller hips and busts – although significantly ano-rexics do not want their breasts to shrink – and Miss World weighs progressively less each year.

'Shameful', cry some, but the parades of emaciated female beauties continue, and young women still slavishly copy the fashion they believe will increase their sexual attraction. A great many devote themselves obsessively to this pursuit. But it is not so easy for the adolescent female, especially when she is intelligent, who comes from a family where competition is encouraged and academic suc-cess and professional achievement applauded. All too often she finds herself in a cleft stick. It is painfully hard for her to mix work and sex. Success in her exams requires long hours alone with her books. While her friends, less concerned with their scholastic results, spend time on their looks and men, the potential anorexic is tied compulsively to her studies. She is fearful of doing less well than she should. 'I may fail', she wails repeatedly, and she cannot be persuaded otherwise by her family or teachers, however confident they are in her; what she really means is that she may fail herself, and not come up to her own high standards. She casts all thoughts to do with her looks, men and sexual enjoyment from her, although occasionally she looks longingly at her erstwhile friends who seem so happy and carefree. But by now she is gripped by the fear of failing generally and even the idea of a boyfriend is too ambitious to contemplate: no man will like her for long and a relationship must end in failure.

The successful woman portrayed by the media is not only attrac-tive and sexually desirable, and able to take a husband and have children if she wishes, but top-class as a student and in her career. The anorexic quails and trembles when she looks not only at the competition facing her, but at the bias and inequality of opportunity that still hampers ambitious, able women, male protestation notwithstanding. The obstacles ahead look insurmountable. The message that thinness is the pointer to success sounds ever louder. For the anorexic, thinness is her only hope – but in reality it is her doom, representing as it does her rejection of the traditional feminine role.

Reinforcing and prolonging factors

The natural course of anorexia nervosa is towards recovery, despite a reputation for relapsing. The majority of anorexics eventually get better, usually without much medical intervention. But some wobble up and down, seemingly recovering and then relapsing; and a few never recover and sink into chronicity, miserable, frozen, emaciated, forever preoccupied with what they may and may not eat. There are several reasons for this.

Emaciation itself has a relapsing effect; it narrows the mind, inhibits and distorts conceptual thinking and self-perception, and encourages depression and apathy. This is why therapists are often so insistent on restoring weight quickly; psychotherapy, to be useful, requires a reasonable weight.

Many teenage anorexics are immature. Some are exceptionally late in reaching puberty, and are backward compared with their peers in their psychosexual and social development; childlike needs linger and they are slow to develop adult relationships, with their mutual give-and-take with either sex; such girls cling for protection to parents or their substitutes, unwilling to take responsibility for themselves. This dependence on their families, often the product of a naturally slow maturation, and over-protective family influences, gradually lessens as social life widens and outside influences become more important; only when parental influences are strongly prohibitive does this fail to occur.

When anorexia nervosa develops against such a background and the anorexic's difficulties are revealed to the family, she is then in a position to loosen her ties with her parents and strive for her autonomy. Sheila MacLeod sees her anorexia nervosa as a life saver: without the illness, she believes, she would have been nothing. But some families continue to maintain a strong protective shell and the anorexic fails to break free; her problems may be acknowledged but nothing is done about them, no ally comes to her aid, no therapist gives her the requisite courage and support to push for freedom, and she sinks into chronicity and despair. The longer anorexia nervosa persists the more demoralized the individual becomes and the less chance there is of recovery, of gaining her autonomy. The 20 year old who has been ill since 16 still has a good potential to recover. She has lost important years but once she can begin to free herself and stand on her own feet, she will soon acquire the social skills and confidence that are needed for her recovery to proceed unabated. But for a 28 year old, anorexic for 10 years or more, there is a less optimistic, although certainly not hopeless future; difficult as it is to break free after so many lost years and join the world as an adult, with determination and help it is possible.

Chapter 3

Clinical Aspects

Anorexia nervosa presents in a number of ways, but the cardinal feature is always a relentless, tenacious pursuit of thinness. The anorexic celebrates the loss of weight and mourns when she gains.

The teenager with anorexia nervosa usually loses weight through dieting and increased exercise alone. Some, dissatisfied with the rate of their progress, boost the speed of loss by abusing laxatives. Others, less disciplined and liable to give way to a stupendous binge, resort to vomiting. Strict abstainers often regard vomiting with abhorrence, although some occasionally try half-heartedly and in the end unsuccessfully to make themselves sick.

Sometimes the bursts of irresistible appetite are so frequent that the non-vomiter despairs. Laxatives alone, she feels, are not enough and she develops an ever more chaotic eating pattern; days of almost total starvation alternate with ravenous gorging. This is *bulimarexia* which in time may develop into bulimia nervosa.

Anorexia nervosa can develop like a bolt from the blue, unheralded and unexpected by the family, but more often it emerges slowly from a seemingly normal attempt to diet. First-born and youngest children are slightly more prone to develop the condition. They may be tall or short, blonde or brunette, nearly always physically attractive and intelligent, and usually from middle-class, Protestant, Catholic or Jewish families. It used to be unusual among ethnic minorities, but is steadily becoming less so as these families absorb Western attitudes and ideas, and become more affluent and academically ambitious for their children.

Typically the anorexic is a 'good girl' who has never seriously rebelled and always tried to succeed and please her parents and other important adults. At school she is in the top half of the class.

She usually has one, at most two close friends on whom she depends; the loss of such a friend, through change of schools or a quarrel, sometimes sparks off anorexia. She tends to be introverted and sensitive. She gives her parents no trouble, and consequently neither one sees the storm gathering beneath the surface.

The first signs may be perceived by her parents as outrageous behaviour but in truth she is merely copying her school friends; showing an interest in boys, going to parties and coming back late, entering pubs and drinking shandy with a group of companions, spending less time on her school work, smoking cigarettes, even marijuana, in her bedroom. Her parents are bewildered and threaten to impose sanctions, and treat her like a small child. She is upset by the anger and concern she has aroused and begins to feel bad and unlovable. She turns herself inside out, suppresses her new-found emotions and controls herself in the way the family expect. She withdraws from her friends, refuses invitations and concentrates on her work.

More often her early rebellion takes a minor form; mild rudeness and reluctance always to do the right thing. Or, not infrequently, it is bypassed altogether, and the parents notice that their daughter is working harder than before, has come top of her form, and is a model of good manners and behaviour. She rarely sees her friends outside school hours, become more dependent on her mother, and prefers the company of her parents' friends; she shows little or no interest in the opposite sex unless it be a much older, fatherly man she has long known, and whom she worships from afar.

Vegetarianism, occasionally total but usually limited to the exclusion of red meat, is sometimes adopted a year or more before the start of strict dieting. This seems to reflect fears of her developing aggressive instincts, and it rarely persists after anorexia nervosa has been resolved.

About a third of anorexics are initially overweight, although rarely to a marked degree. Often this is because they have eaten for comfort, to counteract their growing discontent and anxiety. Jessica

(1.68m; 5'6") weighed 62 kg (9¾ stone) at fourteen. She then began to eat compulsively between meals and, 2 years later, when anorexia nervosa developed, she weighed nearly 76 kg (12 stone).

Most adolescent girls diet at some time, whatever their weight, and many do so repeatedly. Typically they lose a few pounds, their determination slackens, and they give way to their appetite. The anorexic has, more often than not, experienced this, but this time there is no failure, and soon she is losing weight steadily. She weighs herself daily, often several times a day, and is elated by the steady fall. Unlike past attempts, her success spurs her to diet ever more strictly; she cuts out all fats and carbohydrates until she is subsisting on a few lettuce leaves and a tomato and a small plate of dry cereal or a yoghurt, and endless cups of black coffee, providing a mere 300 or 400 calories a day; rarely, fluids are restricted. Her mind circles endlessly around food and diet. She reads avidly everything she encounters on food and dieting and she is fascinated by articles on cooking. Not only does she read about the subject, but many anorexics turn themselves into full-time cooks and insist on cooking for the family; some literally turn their mother out of the kitchen. Huge meals are produced which, the anorexic insists, must be completely consumed: the smallest scrap left on the family's plates is seen in terms of rejection, and noisy, angry scenes ensue. Needless to say, the anorexic eats almost nothing, and sits enthralled by the masticatory efforts of the family. At that moment the family is beholden to her. Unchecked the anorexic soon becomes the tyrant of the kitchen and meal table.

At first her parents are encouraging. They help her with her diet and applaud her weight loss. But sooner or later they begin to have misgivings. She has already passed the target she set herself. Why does she not stop, or at least modify the diet? The anorexic agrees with them; she will eat more. But in fact this previously scrupulously truthful girl now begins to lie and deceive. She pretends she has eaten a huge school lunch, she is not hungry at supper because she had cakes or chocolate at teatime, and so on. She tries to absent herself from family meals, and when forced to eat with her parents she dawdles, cuts her food into tiny pieces which she chews very slowly, pushes the food to the edge of the plate and surreptitiously disposes of it to the dog, or with remarkable sleight of hand, transfers it to bags which she hides about her body.

As her parents become increasingly upset and attempt to re-establish their authority, so their daughter becomes more deceitful and obstinate. The child who was so good cannot now be trusted. Rows break out. Her family, which was outwardly so united and peaceful, now continually bicker and disagree.

The anorexic, despite her sense of triumph, is increasingly anxious; she is isolated and cut off from her parents. 'I can't talk to my mother, or father', she declares, meaning in a roundabout way that she no longer feels loved by them. But the elation that accompanies every loss of weight, the joy released by knowing that she is in control of her appetite and body quickly sweeps such feelings aside. She has little time to spare for the family, even at mealtimes, for almost every waking moment is occupied by thoughts of further weight loss and thinness.

Only much later when she begins to realize that the thinness she seeks exists only in her mind, not in reality, is her elation eroded by doubts and fears. Fleetingly at first she recognizes that the thinness she seeks is only possible in death. Very few anorexics choose death. The vast majority want life.

To increase her loss of weight the anorexic exercises at every spare moment. Her energy is phenomenal. It is as though her mental elation keeps the body continually wound up and taut. She is awake and jogging or bicycling soon after dawn. At other times, or if the weather is inclement, she exercises furiously in her room, sometimes with ostentatious noisiness. A few acquire bizarre habits such as sleeping without blankets beside an open window in winter, believing that the violent shivering and sleeplessness enhance weight loss, deriving masochistic satisfaction from the painful cold. But such behaviour is rare and is an ominous prognostic sign.

Drugs are also used to aid slimming, although slimming pills themselves – drugs to suppress appetite – are now extremely dif-ficult for a young woman to obtain on prescription. But laxatives are freely available and many anorexics dose themselves regularly with them. Those whose strict dieting is interrupted by bouts of bulimia are particularly likely to abuse laxatives. Diuretics are also employed, again mainly by those who binge. They do not, of course, lower body mass as such, but they temporarily reduce the fluid in the body and so give the anorexic the satisfaction, even though short lived and illusory, of seeing her weight drop.

Food is vomited before most of it can be absorbed by many anorexics who binge, and by most people with bulimia nervosa. Vomiting is a remarkably easy process, and can often be carried out reflexly, without effort. But some find it more difficult and need to fill their stomachs with water first, while others have to thrust a finger or spoon handle down their throat. The knowledge that food can be safely ejected lessens the anorexic's fear that she may eat too much and become fat. Even a vast binge, depressing as it is, can be tolerated without fear, for the relief and satisfaction that follow vomiting are enormous. It is the satisfaction felt at the start of a binge – the pleasure of the first few mouthfuls – together with the intense relief that succeeds vomiting that make this pattern so difficult to alter.

The vomiter is ashamed of her behaviour and usually hides it from everyone; some continue to practise it for years without parents or spouse guessing. When the anorexic leaves traces of vomit on the lavatory seat or wash-basin, she is surely appealing for help and wishing to communicate her distress. The combination of vomiting and laxatives, and especially with diuretic abuse, is highly dangerous; the consequent loss of electrolytes can cause the heart suddenly to stop.

Warning the anorexic of the dangers of abusing her body can occasionally cause her to stop or lessen the practice, but although she may be alarmed the compelling drive towards thinness and fear of increasing weight are usually too fierce for her to change her behaviour. Her perception of her *body image*, of the shape of her body, especially below the waist, is grossly distorted. An anorexic of skeletal appearance steadfastly maintains that she is too fat (although when relaxed she may admit she *feels* rather than sees she is too fat, and she knows at heart that she is too thin despite the desire to be even thinner). Indeed she is ashamed to display her thinness and reluctant to appear on a beach in a swim-suit. Her usual dress is a flowing kaftan, or baggy clothing that disguises her body. The distortion of her body perception increases in proportion to her emaciation. At a reasonable weight the anorexic is no more likely to see herself fatter than she really is than another young woman. Most women today are so figure-conscious that, in terms of averages, it is normal to have a distorted body image.

Meanwhile the anorexic's eating habits are liable to become progressively more eccentric. She may demand to eat alone in her room. Or, if she continues to eat with the family she insists on cooking, or having cooked, her own diet, exactly the same each day in content and amount. Carol, for instance, always had a slice of boiled breast of chicken and four spoonfuls of cabbage for dinner. Occasionally, and this occurs only among those who are liable to binge, the anorexic raids the dustbin or waste bin and consumes everything edible there – human, canine and feline leftovers – however foul. Such behaviour more often than not occurs at night after the family has gone to bed; they may be woken by the noise. The anorexic, convinced she is rejected, feels permitted to eat food rejected by her family (she never eats out of neighbours' dustbins), the dirtier the better. Like some mystic of old where gluttony represented spiritual death, she satiates herself on filth, doing penance even as she eats. This is usually a short-lived episode; almost, it seems, a symbolic suicide, coinciding with the anorexic's lowest estimate of her worth. Subsequently she begins to return to a more realistic view of herself.

A 'capricious or depraved' appetite was often a feature of chlorosis, so prevalent in the nineteenth century, but this was more for 'dry and tasty' food, something that could be chewed and preferably cracked. One physician of the early eighteenth century believed there were few young women who did not chew rice or unground coffee; and more rarely salt, mortar, chalk, cinders and sealing wax.

A feature of anorexia nervosa sometimes associated with episodes of bingeing is shoplifting. It begins with sweets and other foodstuffs, often but by no means always because the anorexic cannot afford the food for her binges. There is invariably a compulsive element behind the thieving, which again reflects the anorexic's feelings that she is bad and excluded from her society, and a subconscious wish to be caught and punished is often apparent. They neglect the simplest precautions to avoid detection. In time stealing may widen to include jewellery and clothing of a kind to enhance female attractiveness; analogous perhaps to the child dressing up and masquerading, as in charades, as a beautiful woman. Significantly, the anorexic does not steal such objects as books, or unfeminine apparel like winter vests.

Menstruation stops in anorexia nervosa (in a small number the illness begins before the anorexic has reached the menarche). Cessation is usually abrupt and coincides with the onset of dieting, but may date from some months earlier. Amenorrhoea is not therefore usually secondary to loss of weight, but must be caused by still unknown changes in the brain, especially in the hypothalamus, where feeding 'centres' are placed, and which has close connections with the anterior pituitary gland. Occasionally menstruation continues after the start of anorexia nervosa for a variable time, even a year or more, but becomes increasingly sparse and irregular and finally stops. It is the older age of onset anorexic who shows this pattern. Loss of weight in itself upsets menstruation and when considerable stops it altogether, so that even if the original emotional cause of amenorrhoea no longer exists, menstruation will not resume until weight returns to near normal. Some patients then resume their periods immediately, but many have to wait months, a few even years, before menstruation returns.

Most anorexics are at first pleased when menstruation stops, and a few chronic anorexics continue to be so. But after 6 months or a year the majority begin to worry that absence of menstruation means infertility, and seek reassurance that this is not so. Beneath their fears of becoming adult women, responsible for themselves, is a strong wish to have children and become 'good mothers'.

A number of bodily changes accompany starvation. The pulse slows and blood pressure drops. Oedema may develop with swelling of the feet and eyelids; this is sometimes seen, too, when weight is regained too quickly. Lanugo hair – fine and downy, like a babe's – appears over the back, limbs and sides of the face. The skin becomes dry and rough and the colour muddy, mottled with red and purple patches in cold weather, especially the hands and face. Sometimes the palms, soles and area around the nose become orange coloured, and this is more likely when large amounts of raw carrots are consumed. Constipation is usual and all too often treated with laxatives. Natural homeostatic mechanisms for controlling body temperature become inefficient, and this drops; the anorexic is gripped by a paralysing sense of cold, even on the warmest days. The gastrointestinal system functions erratically, hardly surprising with the strange diet it receives, together with purging and vomiting. The stomach empties slowly; consequently, the anorexic quickly feels full. But if and when she binges she is often oblivious to discomfort until a huge amount has been eaten. Then she becomes unpleasantly hot, sweaty and faint.

There are widespread hormonal disturbances in established anorexia nervosa; the thyroid, adrenal and sex glands are all affected, but these apparent abnormalities are the direct result of starvation and glandular activity returns to normal when weight is regained.

The anorexic's mood, which in the early days of dieting often borders on the ecstatic, gradually gives way to depression, deepening as the condition persists. To live in order to diet, to reach for an idealized state of thinness, to be continually threatened in the mind by gluttony and the possibility of becoming fat, is indeed a hellish state. The mind is never at peace and the anorexic can never allow her body to rest; however tired she must push herself to be active. She can tell no one of her misery, for no one comprehends. She herself does not understand why she is compelled to behave thus. In sympathetic surroundings she can sometimes bring herself to admit that her behaviour is absurd but when food appears anxieties flood back and the mental barriers return. She continues to smile at the world and deny that anything is amiss. But behind the clown-like disguise is deep despair.

Obsessional rituals grow. She can take hours to wash and dress and prepare herself to go out. She gets up at dawn to ensure she has enough time for whatever has to be done. In any case she is unable to sleep for more than a few hours at a stretch. Her concentration is impaired for her thoughts constantly return to weight and food. The days are endless and yet all too short. Her isolation feels complete, yet at heart she longs to break out of her prison and escape into the world. Hope continues for years. Only when this finally goes does she turn to suicide.

Chapter 4

Treatment

The patient with anorexia nervosa usually denies she is ill and rejects treatment. Indeed, the idea of seeking to put on weight is too frightening to contemplate; and the anorexic initially perceives the doctor as threatening, not offering help. She usually comes for medical advice at her parents' or spouse's insistence and is, on the surface at least, uncooperative and even hostile. What is the doctor to do, faced with an emaciated adolescent whose weight loss is not due to any organic disease but to her obstinate and seemingly unreasonable refusal to eat enough? How is he or she to respond to anxious relatives demanding that he take drastic action and restore the anorexic's weight? The easiest course perhaps is to threaten the patient, to be coercive: you must eat, you must put on weight, otherwise you will come into hospital. But such an approach is doomed from the start. Coercion should never be used. If the anorexic is to be helped she must co-operate in the treatment, and that requires trust in the therapist and a say in what happens to her; in other words, to accept some responsibility for herself. If all control is taken from her she will certainly put on weight, but the chances are that she will lose it again once she regains her freedom. Anorexia nervosa – except for those mild episodes lasting 6–9 months, so common in adolescence and the early twenties, which require and receive little or no treatment – is long lasting; 2 or 3 years at least and even after apparent recovery the ex-anorexic is prone to relapse.

It is doubtful whether any one type of treatment is superior to another. In practice they are all used in various combinations. What matters above all else is the quality of the relationship that builds up between the anorexic and therapist. Not everyone has the temperament and understanding to cope with such patients. The inpatient's refusal to eat can arouse considerable anger and aggression in doctors and nurses. Conversely a doctor or nurse may identify with the anorexic and then collude with her and encourage her resistance and subterfuges.

Weight gain is frequently slow, but is sometimes extraordinarily fast when the anorexic eats with the sole purpose of reaching her weight target and leaving hospital – and then rapidly ridding herself of the weight. It is often difficult not to lose patience and threaten sanctions, signs to the anorexic that she is very much in control and that empathy is poor.

Some authorities doubt the value of treatment, apart from short-term critical periods when weight is dangerously low, the eating pattern chaotic, or depression is severe. They question whether treatment alters the natural course of the illness. We ourselves believe that admission to hospital is usually necessary at critical periods, but we also recognize that treatment can help a patient recover sooner than she would otherwise do; build up her self-confidence and give support, break a vicious circle at home that is perpetuating anorexic behaviour, and restore bodily functions to normal. But with others, especially chronic anorexia nervosa, treatment provides support only.

This sounds unduly pessimistic, and we must emphasize that the natural course of anorexia nervosa is towards recovery, *provided* the patient is not trapped within her family and has freedom to develop her personality.

Whether it is the family doctor or specialist who first sees the anorexic, the initial consultation is of immense importance, for it may well determine her reaction to any treatment. The girl is interviewed on her own at first. Her relatives, alone or with her, depending on the girl's inclinations, are seen together afterwards.

The doctor's first task is put the patient at ease and allay her anxieties; he must be sympathetic and show that he understands her fears and anorexic behaviour. She may admit that, terrified as she is of her greed and becoming fat, she is also apprehensive that her dieting is out of control; she wants to be thinner, yet she cannot bear her mother's anguish. She is encouraged to talk about herself, her friends and interests, ambitions and achievements, and a picture of her personality constructed. The character of other members of the family, the structure of the family, and how each one characteristically behaves are explored. If it seems appropriate, the doctor suggests possible links between problems that have been exposed and her attitudes to her weight and eating.

Future treatment is then discussed. The doctor emphasizes that he sees the anorexic's eating difficulties – accepted as very real to her – as caused by, and covering up, deeper problems related to growing up; for example, self-confidence and autonomy. All the same, he adds, it is important for treatment to be effective that she regain a reasonable weight. He suggests a low normal weight for her height which, after some haggling and reassurance that she will not go on gaining, she usually accepts.

The vast majority of anorexics are treated as outpatients. Only when a patient is dangerously emaciated, thin and seemingly incapable of gaining weight, in a mentally abnormal state through malnutrition, and occasionally when the home situation has become too difficult for her to cope there, is inpatient treatment necessary.

Methods of treatment

Psychotherapy

Psychotherapy, aimed at increasing the anorexic's sense of autonomy and self-confidence, is an essential ingredient. Therapist and patient meet together once or twice a week for an hour at a time and explore her difficulties and fears, especially those relating to adult relationships and responsibilities, and anxieties over loosening family ties. Feminist views that anorexia nervosa is culturally conditioned, that society's expectations of women as slim and self-sacrificing have to be changed, are discussed and can be linked to parental attitudes.

The results of psychotherapy must be seen from a long-term

point of view. It takes time for the anorexic to build up deep trust in the therapist and feel that she is liked and accepted for her own sake rather than what she does. The therapist becomes a second parent, on whom for a time the anorexic depends. She is encouraged to widen her life, to experiment and take social risks, and gradually take responsibility for herself.

Group psychotherapy

A group of 7 or 8 patients who meet for 1½ hours at a time under the direction of a therapist is obviously a more economical form of treatment. One or two anorexics can be included in a general group, but larger numbers are too difficult to handle and adversely affect the group's general progress. Older anorexics, especially those married or living with a sexual partner, benefit more than adolescents. There is of course no reason why individual and group psychotherapy should not be combined.

In an Occupational Therapy Department, mainly concerned with inpatients although an anorexic can attend as an outpatient several days a week, *play therapy* is a useful addendum to psychotherapy. The anorexic plays the mother or child say, in a family quarrel or celebration, or a scene with her peers, and in the process faces emotions that have so far been suppressed.

Projective art techniques also aim to bring out strong latent feelings, which are subsequently discussed in group or individual psychotherapy.

Family therapy

The aim of family therapy is to explore the attitudes and behaviour of the family and how its members are reacting to the eating disorder. Salvador Minuchin and his colleagues in the USA have published much on this therapy and formulated theories about families where anorexia nervosa exists: they see the condition as a family rather than an individual's disease.

The treatment ideally includes all the family who are closely concerned with the anorexic; obviously the parents or spouse, and if possible siblings, although in practice the latter may be unwilling to attend. The patient and her family and therapist (there can be more than one present) meet as a group for about 1½ hours, and the ways they relate and react to one another are observed and commented upon, including their possible significance in generating anorexia nervosa. A more open approach within the family to disagreements is encouraged, together with greater understanding and tolerance for each individual's opinions and attitudes.

The therapist may actively encourage controversy, or remain comparatively passive and restrict himself to useful comments and interpretations. He needs to be mature as well as skilled. It is all too easy to leave mother or father or a spouse feeling that he or she is entirely responsible for the trouble, hostile to the therapist and angry with the anorexic. If anyone in the family group feels he or she is being held to blame, the matter must be recognized and brought into the open by the therapist. Blame is invariably destructive to progress.

The therapist should not hesitate to offer advice to the family on how to react to the anorexic's eating behaviour. It is extremely difficult for parents to sit beside their daughter at mealtimes and watch her picking and poking at food or chewing a tiny morsel after everyone has finished, and not become exasperated, yet knowing that they are unable to force the girl to eat. One principle has to be accepted by every family member: the anorexic must be given, and accept, full responsibility for what she eats and the consequences of failing to eat enough to maintain weight. Once this happens pressure in the family, especially at mealtimes, lessens. It becomes possible for mother and daughter to discuss food and weight and devise ways and means of reducing the anorexic's anxieties; and for both to recognize the emotional problems behind them.

Cognitive therapy

Cognitive therapy simply means attempting to get the anorexic to think in a different way, particularly about weight and food. Instead of thinking that every mouthful of food turns to fat she tries to think that every mouthful gives her mental energy; instead of saying to herself 'I am greedy, if I eat one bar of chocolate I shall go on and consume twenty', she repeats, 'One bar of chocolate will be lovely and give me all the enjoyment I need'. When she is reluctant to go out because 'no one likes me', she tells herself, 'I am likeable'. This somewhat simplified method depends, like all psychotherapy and behaviour therapy (of which it is a branch) on a trusted, admired therapist. Therapeutic success, whatever the treatment, rests ultimately on a strong positive transference (i.e. recreating feelings of love and trust, which go back to childhood).

Behaviour therapy

There are numerous behaviour modification techniques, aimed at altering the anorexic's behaviour, without exploring underlying psychological causes. Desirable behaviour is rewarded, undesirable 'punished'. For instance, on first coming into hospital the anorexic may be confined to bed – in some hospitals she is isolated in a single room – until she has gained say 3 kg (6½ lb), a figure agreed with her in advance. On the way to this target successive gains of weight are rewarded by such privileges as having a bath, using the lavatory instead of a bedpan, making telephone calls and having visitors. When up and about she is allowed outside the hospital, is unsupervised at mealtimes, and so on as prizes.

We used these techniques at first, but have gradually abandoned them. We believe they encourage childlike dependence, and the concept of 'good girl' which is obviously counterproductive. On the other hand, it is often a relief for the anorexic to spend some days in bed when she begins inpatient treatment. She is too frightened to assume any responsibility for herself and her eating, and bed rest gives her time to reorganize herself and collect her thoughts; if she understands this she does not see bed as a punishment.

Relaxation classes, which include hypnotherapy and hydrotherapy, are combined with positive thinking about eating, and are useful especially in the later stages of treatment.

Physical treatment

At one time drugs were extensively used, but it is now generally accepted that they have little part to play in treatment. Depression is common in older, and especially chronic anorexics and an antidepressant can be helpful there. Hypnotics at night are best avoided unless insomnia persists, when they can be given for a week or so. As weight improves so does sleep. Major tranquillizers like chlorpromazine are now given only to inpatients in hospitals where skilled nursing is in short supply and weight gain is slow. In large doses they lower the anorexic's resistance to eating, and enhance weight gain. Their great disadvantage is that they make the patient drowsy, which she sometimes bitterly resents, and they are liable to have serious side-effects. The therapist may have to weigh these disadvantages against the dangers of allowing starvation to continue.

In the past a small dose of insulin was commonly injected before meals, on the grounds that this stimulates appetite. It was more dangerous than helpful and is rarely used today. There are no drugs that can make a resistant anorexic eat without external pressure and encouragement.

There is no place for ECT (electroshock) today except *possibly* as a life-saving measure. The same can be said about tube feeding, which is a barbaric act and an admission of therapeutic despair. It is better to feed the emaciated anorexic intravenously with a balanced mixture of electrolytes and calorific foods if all else fails.

Diet

After having dieted, perhaps severely for many months, the anorexic must reverse the trend slowly. A light bland diet may be all that the emaciated girl can cope with at first. Too much or too heavy a meal is apt to cause involuntary vomiting. Gradually the amount of food is increased and after 10 or 14 days the anorexic should, ideally, be eating a diet of between 3000 and 4000 calories a day; four regular meals and snacks in between and at bedtime. The anorexic's fads should be respected; for instance she may be a vegetarian, and the dietician should take this into account.

It is always necessary to keep in mind the anorexic's terror of growing fat. She and the therapist agree on a weight target at the start of treatment and it is important that the therapist allays her fears that she will go on gaining beyond that. At the same time of course he must point to the deeper meaning of her fears and the reasons for the anorexia.

Weight increases irregularly and it is well to weigh the patient not more than once every 3 days. A graph can be kept over her bed of the weighings, which will help to accustom her to each new rise. Once she has reached her target, one weighing a week or fortnight is quite enough. Losses or unexpected gains need to be explained and the reasons understood. Gradually, with success, the anorexic's anxiety fades.

Chapter 5

Anorexics and Partners

Anorexics of older age of onset develop the same signs, symptoms and eating problems as adolescent patients. Some, perhaps 20 per cent of those seen, are really suffering from chronic anorexia nervosa. The woman was anorexic when she married or began to live with her man, either a strict dieter or alternating starvation with binges and vomiting. When living at home with her parents she and her mother were constantly at loggerheads. She views marriage as an escape to a haven of peace and security; the husband as the perfect parent figure, loving and caring for her without stint.

The man who married such a wife is himself playing at marriage and is rarely mature enough to accept the give and take of an adult relationship. He is attracted by the idea of looking after a frail, dependent wife, who needs him in order to survive.

At first, away from the parental home, she improves in mood, although her fear of giving way to greed remains strong. But gradually dissatisfaction stirs below the surface. Her husband is unadventurous and unassertive, he rarely makes love to her, and she begins to feel unloved and unlovable, a failure as a wife. He treats her as a child and expects her to behave as he wants. Her fears and reluctance to eat increase as she suppresses her growing resentment and depression, and she starts to lose weight.

Many of these older patients, however, are seemingly well and of normal weight when they marry, and are certainly well when they become engaged. However, some have had an episode of anorexia nervosa during adolescence from which they apparently recovered and resumed menstruation. But neurotic conflicts and fears remained; marriage occurred before the woman was psychologically ready to cope and brought on a relapse. Although the husband of such an anorexic tends to be less passive and more mature than the one described above, sooner or later he fails to satisfy his wife's need for love and closeness; resentment and insecurity build up and rekindle the anorexic's fears of herself and her weight.

Sometimes, especially when a husband is well balanced and gives his wife the support and reassurance she requires without her becoming overdependent on him, the marriage goes well for a time. Then some event occurs, say a pregnancy, or a minor peccadillo on the part of the husband is discovered, which causes the wife's insecurity to surge to the surface and pushes her towards anorexia nervosa.

A vicious circle readily forms. The more emaciated his wife becomes the less desirable sexually she is to her husband. He feels aggrieved at her incomprehensible behaviour and at what she is doing to herself. As she loses weight so she grows ever more childlike and deceptive; she pretends to eat, cooks her husband huge meals which she watches him eat and insists on his finishing, and perhaps vomits in secret. A large void opens between the couple.

Many of these marriages have characteristics in common with the anorexic's family. The couple are over-involved with one another, conflicts are ignored and never openly aired, and husband and wife fail to adapt and change their attitudes to one another. The couple sometimes allows the situation to drift for years and no one intervenes. The husband is afraid of being blamed, suspects that he is at fault and yet does not understand in what way. But more often than not, if the husband fails to act his parents or in-laws intervene, or his wife's general practitioner lays down the law and insists she see a specialist.

Treatment is, in essence, no different from that of younger patients. Weight has to be restored, but unless the anorexic is dangerously thin hospital is best avoided. The first priority is to recognize the marital problem and begin therapy with the couple together. At the same time the anorexic needs individual psychotherapy, to look at her underlying fears and behaviour more closely. She feels a failure as a wife and blames herself for not pleasing her husband; she must come to see that she has needs, just as much as her husband, and that a good marriage requires continual compromise and adaptation by each partner. It is sometimes said that anorexics are afraid of sex. This is a misleading idea, and the vast majority enjoy making love – which is how they see the act. It is when they sense they are unattractive and unwanted by their husbands that neurotic fears are stirred. Some are frightened of conception, not so much because of possible pain or injury in childbirth, but from fear they may harm or damage the child in some way and fail to be good mothers. All these anxieties need to be discussed in depth.

The husband also needs psychotherapeutic help, not only to understand his wife and her behaviour but to recognize where his own anxieties lie, and that some of his expectations of marriage and his view of his wife are perhaps unreasonable.

When the couple are realistic and determined and quick to see what has gone wrong, the vicious circle at home is broken and anorexia nervosa disappears, although it may take a year or more before recovery is full. In other cases the anorexic's weight improves, but the marriage remains indifferent. Sometimes the couple separate or divorce, usually on the instigation of the husband. All too often the anorexic is deeply distressed by such a move and demoralized to the extent of returning to her parents' home. She seldom takes the initiative and rarely declares her independence. Psychotherapy is essential at this stage, not only in a supportive sense, but to encourage her to throw excessive caution to the winds, widen her life and, for the first time, accept responsibility for herself.

Chapter 6

Male Anorexia Nervosa

Richard Morton, in his *Treatise of Consumption*, written in 1698, described two cases of what he called 'nervous atrophy', who clearly suffered from anorexia nervosa. One was a young man of 16, the son of a minister, who while 'studying too hard' became emaciated. He was dispatched from home, forbidden all books and fed large quantities of asses' milk (long regarded as beneficial to invalids), and recovered after 2 years.

About one in every 16 or 20 patients today with anorexia nervosa is male. Like their female counterparts they are intelligent and academically ambitious, and come from middle-class homes, often with one or both parents belonging to a profession. The vulnerable age, when they are most liable to become anorexic, is between 15 and 18, when they are working for important school exams or preparing for university. It can develop in older age groups and in married men, but this is rare and, in our experience, has invariably been preceded by eccentric eating habits in adolescence.

There is no one type of personality specifically associated with male anorexia nervosa. But the majority tend to be quiet and diffident and do not enjoy combative games like soccer or hockey; for sporting activities they are more likely to take up rowing or long-distance running. A description in 1839 of men who developed chlorosis – almost certainly anorexia nervosa under another name – is appropriate: 'the young and delicate of the male sex'.

A male anorexic behaves and thinks much as the female does. He wants be thin and is fearful of his greed and becoming fat, he exercises whenever possible, and spends hours each day thinking of food and diets. He no longer has penile erections, and as his libido fades so his need to masturbate disappears; this is because of the hormonal changes that follow the loss of weight, analogous to the female's cessation of menstruation.

Why is anorexia nervosa so much more likely to affect females? What protects males, and what characterizes those who develop the condition? There are in fact no clear-cut features marking out the young man likely to become anorexic. He can be a single child or one of many, tall or short, well built or slender. He usually has pleasant looks, and his sexual inclinations are heterosexual. He tends to be quiet, reserved, more dependent on his parents than his siblings, and prior to dieting has not rebelled or tried to break away from family ties and traditions. Physical aggression has never appealed to him, although he can be intellectually forceful. It may be that the upsurge of aggression and sexual instincts that develop with puberty alarms him – as it does many – and he tries to restrict his strength and bodily drives through starvation. Other influences must surely be present to push him in this direction, and these can only come from within his family or society.

The male anorexic's family resembles that of his female counterpart; there is a tight interdependence, a tendency to keep tensions out of sight and to deny problems, and parental reluctance to see change in their children. But whereas the fathers of female anorexics are frequently unsure of themselves, and either ineffectual and retiring at home or – the other side of the coin – inclined to be loudly dogmatic, the male anorexic's father is more assertive and, outwardly at least, the leader of the family; although once the surface calm is broken, conflicts between the parents spill into the open.

Just as girls identify naturally with their mother, so youths with their father. Male anorexics are openly hostile towards their mother (or wife) and sometimes refuse to eat or talk with her. Rarely, one encounters the opposite. Then the (usually chronic) anorexic son is inseparable from his mother, mother and son appear to be in continuous harmony; his only act of independence, long accepted by his mother, is his insistence on eating an inadequate diet. Feelings for the father are more mixed; signs of his weakness are seized on and criticized, and capabilities and strengths eulogized, part and parcel of a growing need to distance himself from mother and strengthen his sense of male identity. But his gender is too fragile to be displayed, let alone asserted and, through slimming, he inhibits his sexual and aggressive instincts.

The media may influence this psychological process. Male models are often slim – although not skinny like their female counterparts – and they are presented in advertisements as self-confident, sexy, assertive young men, with the world at their feet. The anorexic's anxiety and envy distort his perception of their shape compared with his: 'I need to be still thinner to be in control of my life – and my world', he thinks, and diets yet more rigorously.

Treatment of the male anorexic differs in no wise from the female, and the outcome is similar.

Chapter 7

Anorexia of Late Onset – Anorexia Tardiva

Many instances of anorexia nervosa occurring in older women have been reported over the last 50 years. John Ryle, a leading British physician before the Second World War, described a condition 'essentially similar' to anorexia nervosa in women aged between 31 and 59 years: 'nervous, voluble, sparrow-like women with sparrows' appetites'. We have treated a number of cases of what we call anorexia tardiva beginning after the age of 40. The older the patient the greater the possibility that weight loss is due to underlying organic or psychotic disease, particularly depression, and these must first be excluded.

Depression of mood is often present in anorexia tardiva and sleep disturbance commonly accompanies emaciation. But the patient with anorexia tardiva has a bird-like alertness which belies serious depression, even though she may complain of exhaustion so great that she 'cannot even lift a spoon' to her mouth and says how intolerable life is. And her resistance to eating has a different quality from the real anorexia of the depressed patient.

Cases of anorexia tardiva divide naturally into two groups: those pursuing thinness at all costs and prepared to use virtually any means available to achieve this and who remain energetic in spite of their emaciated appearance, and those who are anorexic or have 'sparrows' appetites', are afraid to eat much, are usually inactive and spend much of their day lying down or bedridden.

The first type is less common. From her teens or early twenties the woman has usually been faddy, and overconcerned about her weight, and has sometimes had short-lived, untreated episodes of anorexia nervosa. She aggressively denies that there is cause for concern, insists that her weight is reasonable and resists eating. She disposes of food, sometimes vomits, and purges herself with enormous quantities of laxatives. She is also prone to take handfuls of stimulant drugs and diuretics, endless cups of black coffee, and chain smoke. She is constantly on the go and talks incessantly (mainly about herself). She is almost invariably a married woman with a daughter who is a key figure in the condition. She clings possessively to her daughter. When the latter reaches adolescence and seeks to become more independent she begins to behave like a teenager herself, almost it seems competing with her child, dressing inappropriately and making up flamboyantly. Eventually she begins to diet and lose weight and show off her figure ostentatiously.

With this type of patient the husband seems to play an insignificant role. Always henpecked and looked down upon by his wife, he is unable to give much support to his daughter. It is important to encourage the daughter to gain her independence and live a more separate life, even though this may for a time worsen the anorexic's condition.

The second type of anorexia is just as difficult to treat but presents outward differences. The anorexic lies quietly, in bed or on a sofa, alert and conscious of everything that is happening around her. She may ask for tempting foods, but when they arrive take no more than a small mouthful. She resists eating passively, in contrast to the aggression of the first type, rarely vomits and, although she may take laxatives regularly, never does so in large amounts. There is often a lifelong history of minor illness which has caused her frequently to retire to bed.

Her refusal to eat, like the first, is based on resentment felt for one or more members of her family. She is an egocentric woman who has always needed to be the centre of attention, and has usually gained it in the past through physical illness of one kind or another. Her anger circles around her husband, whom she criticizes and denigrates. One husband commented that in 30 years of marriage his wife had never given him a day's pleasure; she was always either ill or complaining of feeling ill, and their sexual and social life was virtually non-existent. Had he not believed that she could not exist without him he would have left her long ago!

Within this group is encountered occasionally an anorexic whose children have left home or who is childless or unmarried, living alone with her mother or husband. The same resentful dependence on the person she lives with is apparent. It is when serious illness or death comes to this essential prop that the patient develops anorexia and begins to starve and lose weight.

Although they appear to be bright, these patients are often depressed, feeling they have nothing to live for. Anorexia tardiva seems to represent a suicidal drive, patients simply allowing themselves to wither away and die. Antidepressant treatment is generally unhelpful in these conditions. Only if the patient can be persuaded or cajoled into modifying her attitude to life, and whoever remains in the family is prepared to help, can there be hope of improvement.

Chapter 8

Outcome

Mild forms of anorexia nervosa recover fully within a year or 18 months. Of the more serious cases, those usually seen by psychiatrists or specialist physicians, most are well or improved within 3–4 years. But some remain chaotic eaters, their lives dominated by concern over their weight, and prone to relapses. A few eventually find the endless struggle within themselves intolerable and end their lives.

The probable outcome of any case of anorexia nervosa seen at the beginning is never easy to predict. How well and fully an anorexic recovers depends partly on the quality of her family life – how democratic it is – and particularly on the breadth of her personality; the more outgoing she is, the greater her ability to make and keep friends, the wider her range of interests, the better the outlook. Never mind that she repeatedly relapses after having her weight increased, perhaps in hospital, in the first 2 or 3 years. The condition, once set in motion has, it seems, to run its course and even when treatment does shorten the duration, recovery has still to be measured in years. At the end of 3 years most anorexics are vastly better; after 4 years the majority are virtually back to normal.

How is recovery to be assessed? By now it is apparent that anorexia nervosa is not simply a disorder of weight and to view the outcome in terms of weight only is misleadingly narrow. We believe that assessment of the outcome of any anorexic must include, in addition to her steady weight and attitude to eating, menstruation and psychosexual development, social adaption, work and physical and mental health.

Weight

At the end of 4 years about three-quarters of severe anorexics have regained a normal or satisfactory stable weight. As long as the anorexic is terrified of the consequences of eating, her weight inevitably remains low. If she enters hospital to be fattened she is liable subsequently, unless she is mature enough and on the point of recovery, to lose the acquired weight. She may lose the weight slowly, as the strains of home or of attempting to be independent exert their effects, or rapidly when the young woman has entered hospital under protest and eaten hugely and increased her weight only to leave as soon as possible. These so-called relapses are not cause for scolding or recrimination or foreboding; rather they are pointers to where help is especially needed. Even when the worst seems over, a minor rebuff from a boyfriend, or criticism of her work by her employer can reactivate fears of failure and so upset her equilibrium that she reverts temporarily to the anorexic pattern of thinking and eating. It is here than an understanding therapist can do so much good in reassuring and helping the girl to understand herself and adapt better to future difficulties. A therapist who panics or takes sides with parents and spouse and scolds is of little use to the anorexic.

Understandably, the newly recovered anorexic often continues to fear her gluttony for some months or even years. She counts the calorific value of everything she eats, denies herself treats like ice-cream or cream teas, and checks her weight regularly. About a third become alarmed and depressed when their worst fears are confirmed and their weight rises as they eat compulsively between meals and at bedtime; or at the end of a meal, they follow the food to the kitchen and finish the leftovers. Such splurges of overeating are likely to diminish and stop within 6 months or a year, but sometimes they continue. The anorexic may become overweight, but this is in most cases a temporary phenomenon. Usually she protects herself by restricting her diet after a binge, a cycle that is effective as long as the binges are reasonably infrequent. More often she resorts to vomiting after overeating, or doses herself with quantities of laxative. Not infrequently the two methods are combined. In 1–2 per cent the binges become an established and dominating part of the anorexic's life; she is ashamed of and dreads the binge, and keeps it secret. She learns to hold her weight steady by vomiting or purging; anorexia nervosa gives way to bulimia nervosa.

The small minority who continue to ruminate continuously on the risk of becoming fat and maintain their weight at starvation level endure miserable, narrow lives. They have no joy and zest, no spontaneity, no pleasurable anticipation of the morrow, little or no social life; there is only endless struggle and discomfort to overcome greed and gain illusory control. Their sole satisfaction, and that is short-lived, is derived from the weighing machine and the mirror. The persistence of emaciation ensures maximum distortion of the body image, and increases the anorexic's fears of fatness. In her mind the outline of her skeletal-like pelvis bulges, the matchstick thighs grow huge. Body mechanisms function erratically. The brain settles into a narrow groove which at any time may give way to psychotic thinking or madness. The vicious circle within chronic anorexia nervosa is complete. Recovery is possible only if the anorexic's circumstances can be dramatically changed.

Menstruation and psychosexual development

Menstruation resumes, or starts for the first time, when a biologically satisfactory weight is regained, i.e. around 80 per cent of the ideal body weight. There is often a prolonged delay of up to 2 years between regaining weight and menstruation. Occasionally, particularly when the anorexic is in her twenties or older, menstruation begins at a comparatively low weight, but this is unusual. Most well-covered anorexics are menstruating within 9 months, and certainly within 2 years. A few fail to start. Some are afraid of the implications of menstruation, and need psychological help to relieve fears concerning sexual relationships. Others require treatment with hormones, a contraceptive pill or an antioestrogen drug like clomiphene, to restart the hormonal cycle. It never does to be impatient in this matter, and it is as well to wait for at least a year, and preferably longer, before using these drugs. The individual must be psychologically as well as physically ready for menstruation, otherwise treatment is likely to fail and demoralization ensues.

The return of regular menstruation is a significant milestone; it is usually welcomed, but delight is sometimes tempered by apprehension, which can cause transient loss of weight.

Menstruation does not return when weight remains low, except occasionally when the anorexic regularly takes a contraceptive pill. Few chronic anorexics have a satisfying sexual relationship; when present it is of a distorted nature; a good adult relationship is incompatible with persistent anorexia nervosa. Most recovered anorexics start or resume a sex life shortly before or just after the resumption of menstruation.

Women who develop anorexia nervosa are heterosexual. It is unusual to encounter an anorexic who is homosexual; in such a case we have found the anorexic behaviour to be atypical.

Most anorexics who recover weight and menstruation marry or live with a stable sexual partner. At least two-thirds of them have children; the pregnancy is uneventful and the ex-anorexic usually prefers to breast-feed. Motherhood does not seem to create any unusual problems.

Independence and social activities

Regressive behaviour characterizes those with anorexia nervosa. They are emotionally dependent on parents and cling to them and their homes, fearful of change. A few travel, the younger ones to a kibbutz in Israel, others to living-in jobs in European countries or the antipodes, hoping to achieve freedom. At the best they maintain a reasonable weight, link up with a caring man, and take responsibility for themselves. But they remain vulnerable and liable to relapse into anorexia if circumstances go against them. At worst they collapse, give up eating and in a desperate state are flown home.

Those who recover their weight move away from home and, with increasing self-confidence, lead satisfactory independent lives.

Academic achievement and occupation

An unrealistic fear of not reaching the standards she has set herself in important examinations like GCSEs or 'A' levels often triggers the start of anorexia nervosa. Anxiety begins to build up at the commencement of the academic year, or even in the preceding holidays, and reaches its peak at the time of preliminary or mock tests. When loss of weight is severe, perhaps requiring hospital admission, the examination is likely to be missed; but frequently the girl struggles on with her studies and passes creditably well. Even when she misses a year she often subsequently returns to her studies. A sizeable proportion go on to university, including a number who are still actively anorexic. Some of these drop out of the course, but most obtain a good degree.

Many anorexics are intensely interested in cooking and this pushes them into cordon bleu courses and work in catering. But such work rarely satisfies them for long after they have regained weight, and they branch out into a variety of jobs. Given their intelligence, conscientiousness and loyalty it is not surprising that, even when underweight, they are rarely unemployed.

Anorexics, recovered or otherwise, have a predilection for working in the caring professions; as nurses, doctors, in paramedical jobs, as teachers or social workers. Many do extremely well.

Physical and mental health

Recovered anorexics are physically healthy; their bodies are not adversely and permanently affected by starvation or such habits as purging and vomiting. Nor do chronic anorexics suffer serious disability from their dietary excesses, apart from a vulnerability to bacterial infections, especially pulmonary tuberculosis.

Any illness that occurs at an important formative period, lasts several years and takes the individual out of circulation, isolates her at home and seriously limits her social life, is likely to have repercussions on her psychological state. Once weight is regained, the anorexic must struggle to acquire what she has missed: confidence in social activities, belief in herself, ability to adapt to upsets and disappointments, a work career, friendships with both sexes. These are not gained overnight, and anxiety and depression are apt to develop readily when there are disappointments and setbacks. Transitory setbacks are usually quickly overcome, but persistent anxiety can sometimes develop in social settings, and become severe enough to force her to limit social life seriously. The ex-anorexic now finds that food has been replaced by social avoidance. Such phobias are most likely to develop in the first year or so of recovery. With help, and as self-confidence grows, it will fade.

Psychiatric disabilities are common in chronic anorexia nervosa. Obsessional and compulsive behaviour develops, usually concerning cleanliness and tidiness. Alternatively, hypochondriasis develops, and competes for attention with the preoccupations over food and weight. Depression, alcoholism and drug abuse not infrequently complicate chronic states when binges alternate with starvation, and vomiting and purging are frequent.

Chapter 9

Bulimia Nervosa

The woman with bulimia nervosa (the word comes from the Greek, meaning 'ox hunger') is preoccupied with thoughts of food and weight and frightened of becoming fat. But unlike the anorexic sufferer, she does not rely on willpower to control appetite and maintain a low weight; instead she limits the amount of food absorbed from her stomach and intestines by vomiting or the use of laxatives, alone or in combination. Her unique characteristic is the periodic consumption of huge quantities of food, invariably when alone. She eats until supplies are exhausted or interrupted, or she feels painfully distended; sometimes she has little or no discomfort, as though her stomach were anaesthetized. After such a binge she vomits copiously, often without effort or by putting a finger down her throat, or if this is not her practice she swallows anything between 20 and 100 laxative tablets – Senokot, Ex-lax, Nylax and Dulcolax are popular. More often than not the two purging methods are used together.

Bulimia nervosa was first described as a clinical entity and named in 1979. It has probably occurred whenever and wherever a sophisticated society has existed, among both sexes but predominantly the female. Initially bulimia nervosa was thought to be an extension of anorexia nervosa, gradually evolving from that condition. This is often so, and bulimic behaviour can supplant anorexia after intervals of months or years. But bulimia nervosa can also occur without the anorexic stage, although the mental characteristics of anorexia nervosa are always apparent.

Women, and a few men, with bulimia nervosa are seen frequently by specialists today. The widespread publicity given to the condition by journalists and broadcasters has not only encouraged those who formerly binged and purged in secret to seek help, but led many young women to copy bulimic behaviour and release previously incipient fears and urges.

Once started the bulimic pattern is difficult to break. There is huge satisfaction in taking the first half-dozen bites, although some individuals are so tense and excited when they begin to binge they are barely conscious of their actions, almost as though they are sleepwalking, and feel enormous relief when gorging is terminated by vomiting and all danger of fatness removed.

The bulimic's weight may fluctuate up and down 10 kg (22 lb) or more, depending on the frequency of the binges and effectiveness of purging. Some binge several times a day, others once a week or fortnight only. Many are able to maintain a steady normal weight and hide their actions, so that even their spouse or flat-mate has no suspicion. Others, closer to anorexia nervosa than bulimia, maintain an emaciated state, alternating binges with near-starvation, vomiting after the smallest morsel, and purging themselves several times a week with 100 or more laxative tablets at a time.

The bulimic's attitude to swallowing laxatives is a mixed one. She is relieved to think of the excretory effect on food, of the food being swept from her body. At the same time she dreads, and yet is pleased because it signifies success, the pain and malaise caused by the laxatives and the several hours of diarrhoea that will certainly disrupt her life. At times she fears she is damaging her body by such abuse, but this anxiety is not strong enough to counteract the fear of fatness, and so it continues.

The desperately anxious bulimic, wholly taken up with fears of the shape of her body, will take other drugs, any kind that may help to keep fatness at bay. These will include diuretics, thyroid extracts, and stimulants like caffeine and the no longer easily available amphetamines.

The bulimic binges when she is lonely, anxious and frustrated. Food becomes a substitute for most of the emotions. The bulimic who works is liable to devour food soon after arriving home, provided she is alone and has suitable supplies. She may have had a minor splurge at lunchtime and eaten several chocolate bars and sticky cakes. Having given in once, she decides, she may as well abandon self-control for the rest of the day; as the afternoon wears on she ruminates pleasantly on what food to buy on the way home: sweet biscuits, chocolate, cakes, puddings, the very foods she usually avoids. If she cannot afford them she may be impelled to steal them. She behaves almost as though she were an automaton; although she is aware of her actions she does not fully appreciate the consequences. Only when her appetite is halted by discomfort or food runs out and the binge cycle is completed by purgation, does she really understand what has happened. Then she is engulfed by depression and despair.

For some bulimics, either unmarried or dissatisfied with their husband, the time immediately before bedtime is most tempting. No sooner is she in her night-clothes than she is compelled to go to the kitchen and eat whatever is available. It is as though food is necessary to offset loneliness, or to reduce the anxiety and resentment she feels for her sexual partner. The bulimic housewife, tied to her home and children, is most threatened when she is in the kitchen preparing meals, on her own and often bored. She nibbles and is immediately lost; the piece of pastry is followed by hunks of bread and jam, bowls of cereal and milk, packets of biscuits until, gastronomically exhausted, she vomits and doses herself with Ex-lax before her children return.

The bulimic woman often differs temperamentally from the abstaining anorexic. She is more outgoing and impulsive, more prone to swing quickly from depression to joy and back again. She easily makes friends and acquaintances, and she prefers other people's company to her own; she is uneasy when alone. Bulimia does not necessarily disrupt social activities, and most bulimics can eat normally, their appetite controlled in the presence of others. Altogether she is a warmer, more extroverted individual than the anorexic. But being so strongly affected by emotions she is prone to depression and dramatic gestures such as slashing her wrists and taking overdoses, appeals for help rather than serious suicide attempts. She often looks for stimulants to keep up her spirits and reduce her appetite; strong black coffee may be drunk compulsively and numerous cigarettes smoked. Alcohol is sometimes abused, but the average bulimic is not tempted, partly because of the calories it contains but mainly because it is apt to lower resistance to over-eating.

Married bulimics who keep their feeding habits to themselves, provided their binges are not too frequent, can be happily married on the surface, although guilt and depression borne in isolation take their toll. A binge not only destroys libido but makes the very idea of intercourse repellent. When the spouse shares his wife's secret, she feels able to confess her lapses, and not only is she comforted, but better understanding develops between husband and wife; ultimately the couple may so adapt their life that bulimia is overcome.

Bulimia can cause a number of complications. Frequent vomiting gradually dissolves the enamel of the teeth and discolours and rots them. Hiatus hernia and oesophagitis, producing pain in the chest, develop after years of vomiting. Habitual purging may affect the lower bowel. More serious, the loss of fluids and electrolytes, especially potassium, from vomiting and diarrhoea can bring on epileptic fits, result in a heart attack, and impair the actions of the kidneys.

Treatment

Treatment can be short, simple and successful or complex, time consuming and ineffectual, depending on the strength of the bulimic's personality and her circumstances.

As always the therapist to be of any help must quickly gain the bulimic's confidence and trust; only then will she disclose herself and speak freely about what she is afraid and ashamed of.

The first stage is to analyse her daily routine and highlight the danger periods when she is most likely to binge. She should keep a diary for the next month in which she records her eating pattern, when and what she eats and why. Circumstances and her state of mind before she binges, if and when she day-dreams about food, and her thoughts at the end of a binge cycle should be detailed. Therapist and client can discuss the record and begin to formulate a treatment programme.

Simple measures include at least two regular meals a day, preferably three, amounting to 1600 calories, just sufficient to maintain her weight; she must avoid long periods of starvation which are certain to end in a food orgy. If she lives alone, or with a friend or parents, available food should be kept to a minimum. There should be no puddings, ice-creams or packets of biscuits or pasta in the refrigerator, rather cartons of yoghurts. The larder can also be kept comparatively empty or the door locked.

When the vulnerable time is being alone in her flat, the bulimic should go direct from work to a sports activity and relax through exercise. When she is alone at home she must plan to listen to the radio, watch a television play likely to hold her attention, or immerse herself in a hobby. When she cannot concentrate on any of these and longs to eat she should telephone a friend, preferably one who knows the problem and can listen and advise sympathetically.

Cognitive therapy, attempting to change the bulimic's characteristic thoughts about herself and food helps a few: 'I can eat and enjoy a single Mars bar. I have a normal appetite', she repeats to herself. Numerous behavioural methods, aimed at changing reactions to tempting foods, body image and weight and purging have been devised but none alone is particularly effective.

Individual psychotherapy, giving support and advice, providing an opportunity for confession to the bulimic, provides the vital background to whatever treatment is employed. But it is time consuming and group psychotherapy is often employed instead; eight or ten bulimics meet together with a therapist once or even twice a week for a limited period. Self-help groups have evolved in recent years, some based on the principles of Alcoholics Anonymous. Variable numbers of bulimics meet, confess their transgressions over food, and offer each other support, and discuss anxieties relating to their lives and weight. Some act as 'sponsors' and are agreeable to being telephoned by group members tempted to give way to a binge.

Bulimia nervosa tends to develop after adolescence, and family therapy is then rarely appropriate. But marital therapy, meeting with the bulimic and her sexual partner, can be rewarding. The couple are encouraged to disclose their tensions, resentments and dissatisfactions and trace the possible connection between these and bulimic behaviour. Each strives to adapt to the other's needs, and the measure of success is the absence or steady reduction of bulimic outbursts.

Antidepressant drugs are occasionally helpful when depression is severe and blocks psychotherapeutic progress. Tranquillizers have virtually no place in the treatment of bulimia. They cannot remove the anxiety of the bulimic over her weight, and they are all too easily abused.

Drugs that suppress hunger can be useful for *short* periods and help the bulimic over a bad patch, as much perhaps through their 'pep' action as by reducing hunger. Too large a dose or giving the drug for too long is likely to do more harm than good.

Admission to a specialised unit is necessary when the bulimic's eating pattern and style of life is so chaotic that she cannot hope to control herself and co-operate as an outpatient. In hospital, with skilled help, she learns to eat regularly and gradually resist the temptation to gorge. This may take months, and is only the preliminary to learning to cope with herself and the outside world. A long, close follow-up is essential if the gains are to be not just retained but built upon.

As with all eating disorders, a good prognosis depends on the bulimic being reasonably mature and able to develop a satisfactory relationship with a close friend or partner.

Part Two
Obesity

Chapter 10

How Fat is Too Fat?

Fatness is mainly a matter of how a person feels about herself. This depends on individual circumstances and self-esteem and on current fashion. Despite its present poor image in the West, plumpness is by no means incompatible with fame and approbation. Plato was fat – and held in high regard. Henry VIII, as broad as a playing-card king, was admired for his wit, erudition and majestic person. Cardinal Wolsey, his chancellor, was even fatter, but considered 'very handsome'. In the eighteenth century Dr Johnson, David Garrick and Handel were all extremely stout, while Domenico Scarlatti became so fat he could not cross his hands at the harpsichord. A hundred years ago Oscar Wilde and Henry James were definitely portly, and more recently Hattie Jacques and Hardy of Laurel and Hardy entertained through their size.

While a man's figure, even today, is more or less irrelevant to his success, the shape and build of a woman's body has especial significance. Like food, the female reproductive arrangements are basic to the survival of the species, and a source of recurrent pleasure. When famine was ever-lurking, a well-covered woman was attractively reassuring. In modern Britain it is among the poorest that female fatness is most prevalent. There is a sense that funds, perhaps food, might run low. In ancient Greece, with its wonderful climate, food was abundant, and for health and beauty dietary restraint and herbal purges were used. Socrates' daily dancing was a precursor of the modern slimmers' aerobics craze. In the affluent Rome of the Caesars food was plentiful and the fashionable had to mind their figures. At feasts the vomitorium was an acceptable method of weight control.

In the Middle Ages and throughout the Renaissance the favoured figure for women was the 'reproductive shape' with big hips, thighs and abdomen as portrayed, for example, in the voluptuousness of Rubens', Tintoretto's and Rembrandt's models. During the era of exploration – the fifteenth to seventeenth centuries – trade and a middle class of merchants emerged. Their pride in possessions and 'keeping a good table' prepared the ground both for obesity and anorexia nervosa. The industrial revolution of the nineteenth century meant that more people could acquire wealth without physical labour or lands. Apart from the Dickensian poor there was widespread affluence. Shut out from the professions and without enough marriageable men to go round, Victorian women were in competition. To ensure attracting a husband they improved on nature. Medical advances had made childbirth safer. Now the fashionable figure was not just a baby machine, but exaggerated both bosom and bottom, with a whale-boned constriction at the waist: the mantrap-plus-maternal-promise design. By contrast, men merely had to look substantial.

Women's magazines, then as now, concentrated on food and fashions, but among a handful of intellectuals, the feminist movement began. From these nineteenth century beginnings the liberation of women advanced dramatically – speeded by two world wars.

In general, when there is abundance of food, fashion acclaims the thinnest body as the most beautiful, the most basic diets the healthiest. In the 1920s, when food flowed freely after the First World War, elegant women wore short, straight, unwaisted garments to match their flat-chested figures. Flappers starved to achieve this shape. Augustus John and Picasso were painting narrow, streak-like women. After the Second World War, when the West had 'never had it so good', the reaction to plenty was epitomized by the run-away popularity of Twiggy, a waif-like slip of a model with no hint of potential maternity. The mini-skirt came in, suitable only to the pre-adolescent. Although Twiggy has matured into curves and motherhood, the ideal image still applies. The mini-skirt is back with its message of perpetual youth, while more middle-aged women are seeking hormone replacement rather than accepting the burdens of the menopause; and such movements as Positive Health and vegetarianism make it seem inferior, 'square', unprogressive to be generously built.

Unfortunately, while fashion extols super-slenderness, the average weight-for-height of women in the West has increased during this century. Many are striving for what they will not achieve. Those who are definitely fat are deemed obvious failures or gross non-conformers; a few with anorexia nervosa are over-conformers. They achieve nothing else. In other cultures, other times, the reverse situation applied. Speke, the explorer, looking for the source of the Nile, found a tribe for whom massive obesity was the acme of female beauty. The chief's daughter is described: 'A lass of 16, stark naked before us, sucking at a milk pot, on which her father kept her at work with a rod in his hand'. The Banyankole in East Africa still send their daughters to the fatting house, something like a finishing school. After a year's course the pupils emerge plump, pale and weak. In more than half of non-industrialized societies the preference is for women to be fat by Western standards.

Conformity to fashion and sexual appeal are of compelling importance to women. Men have often exploited this as a means of domination. The obese Banyankole are as handicapped as the Chinese with tiny bound feet or the Victorian ladies, barely able to breathe for tight lacing. The current painful obsession with dieting reflects the ongoing efforts of women to be perfect. Many protest that this is not to attract men, but the wives of successful men are nearly all thin: some to the point of haggardness. Public prejudice against women in particular who are fat is beyond question. Schoolchildren as young as 6 denigrate the fat as 'lazy, sloppy, dirty – and cheats'. Others see them as 'uninfluential, like a mother, unattractive, old, weak'. A group of health workers describe their overweight clients as self-indulgent and suffering from personality problems. Even doctors demand universal slenderness and are frequently unsympathetic to the plight of obese patients, considering them 'weak-willed, ugly and awkward'. Parents are ashamed of plump daughters past puberty, and some exercise unpleasant punitive concern and criticism. In work also, even mild overweight delays promotion for women, while fat housewives may find they are debarred from adopting a child. What is basically a common variant of the human form is treated as some kind of despicable character flaw.

No wonder women are neurotic about their shape. Eighty-five per cent of 18-year-old girl students want to lose weight; 45 per cent of the men want to put it on. In a recent American survey of normal weight women (mean 58 kg; 9st 2lb), 47 per cent saw themselves as too fat, 59 per cent had been actively dieting to reduce in the past month, and 89 per cent wanted to be thinner. Seven times as many men as women thought they were underweight. The women relied mainly on diet to keep their weight in check, while men who wanted to lose preferred to step up their exercise. Conflicts about what and how much to eat have intensified. The technological revolution of the twentieth century has put physical work into decline, including domestically, while every variety of food is available at affordable prices: whether in the country village or city centre. There are pre-prep meal packs, take-aways are ubiquitous, and eating out is commonplace. McDonald's and the pizza places provide for the majority, and various exotic foreign restaurants for the rest. There are also powerful anti-food pressures: television pictures of the victims of earthquake, flood and famine tease the conscience. Distasteful exposés of factory farming methods and alarmist warnings about additives, contamination, pesticides and animal-based foods in particular complete the switch-off of the sensitive appetite. Vegetarianism has become more prominent in the media and gained wide attention.

Nouvelle cuisine is a compromise for some: minuscule portions of 'natural' foods at enormous price. Some dissenting extroverts eat to capacity. Children, willy-nilly dependent on adults for their nutrition, may find they are restricted to 'what is good for you' – with a conscientious mother. The delights of doughnuts, burgers and sausage rolls are denied them, and some children have even been mildly stunted in their growth by over-control.

A woman no longer needs huge hips and a capacious pelvis to produce enough children for some to survive. Competence in the current century means mobility, athleticism, youth and educational attainment: for either sex.

Conclusions

Being too fat is mainly subjective. Being fat is in the eye of the fashion-conscious beholder, and only occasionally a medical matter. It is impossible to imagine a Sumo wrestler considering himself too fleshy, yet agonized complaints of a fat stomach are made by the most skeletal anorexics. Wanting to be thinner is almost universal among Western women. Apart from the small, exceptional group of grossly overweight, the evidence for danger from fatness to life or health is shaky – and for women, negligible. In a recent review of studies and statistics the investigators concluded that the best prospects for a long life included weight somewhat above the average. This cool scientific view contrasts with the avid concern of health and fitness zealots over the slightest upward deviation of weight.

Chapter 11

Who Gets Fat and Why: Physiology

Early Life

Newborn babies with diabetic mothers tend to be big, plump but delicate, due to the high sugar level in their mother's blood. Most of the babies lose their excess fat in the first few months. With normal babies it is noticeable by about day four that individuals differ in the amount of milk they drink. Those who are bottle-fed with over-strong mixtures may take in more nourishment than they need, because they have to drink enough to quench their thirst. These babies put on weight fast, but the situation usually rights itself during the toddler stage.

Genetic effects

Quite apart from some rare hereditary diseases, ordinary fatness frequently runs in families. Average parents have a 1 in 10 chance of having a fat child, but with two plump parents the risk rises to 80 per cent. Family eating habits – like chips with everything – affect a child's weight, but studies on twins and adopted children show a definite genetic influence. Adoptees resemble their natural parents in weight and shape. If only one parent is fat, it does not matter which: it is as relevant to have a fat father as a fat mother. Family fatness usually shows up during childhood, but in some girls it is delayed until the first pregnancy.

Apart from being a target for teasing, childhood fatness is particularly troublesome because of its implications for the future.

There are two types: progressive and reactive. The latter often follows an illness or accident which stops the child running about and burning calories. The situation may be compounded by social circumstances: high-rise flats without gardens, being driven to school because of dangers on the streets, the abolition of compulsory sport, and the lure of passive entertainment by TV. In the more serious, progressive type of fat accumulation, there is an undue increase in the actual number of fat cells, as opposed to a mere increase in size. The greater the number of fat cells the greater the potential for fatness. There are four periods in which fat cells proliferate: before birth, in the first year, at age 7–8 years and finally in early adolescence. After that, while the cells may swell out their number is fixed.

Another childhood feature affecting the future is the tendency of a well-nourished, very active child to develop a large frame and muscles: which in turn predispose to weight gain from forty plus. This is particularly difficult to dislodge. On the other hand, a child who is plump but not energetic does not produce much growth hormone and remains short and podgy.

In most people the rate of metabolism increases after eating, so that rather than being stored as fat, some of the nourishment surplus to current requirements is dissipated as heat: the well-known warm glow after a good meal. The tissue especially adapted for this is brown fat. It is laid down in the weeks just before birth, and accounts for the extraordinary powers of survival of newborn babies abandoned on doorsteps, or exposed after natural disasters: they stay warm. Brown fat, unlike the ordinary white type, is supplied with blood vessels and nerve fibres and is responsive to the body's needs. Much of it is replaced by white fat, especially in females, from the second month onwards. In a substantial proportion of overweight adults the metabolic reaction to a binge is noticeably sluggish. This applies particularly to those who were chubby as children, and it persists after weight loss. These people have no brown fat left.

Size of the problem

Children

In the USA 25 per cent are considered overweight (more than 20 per cent above the expected weight for height, sex and age), about half that number in the UK, and a little less in Australia. Plump little girls outnumber boys 2½:1 up to age 11, rising to 3½:1 from 11–14. From then on the proportions even out. The pound or two put on by many girls at 15–16 does not amount to an excess and disappears as the hormonal rhythm becomes established during the next year. It may account for the term 'puppy fat', with its implication of something harmless and temporary. Unfortunately, time alone does not solve the problem for definitely overweight youngsters.

Adults

In the West women are only half as likely as men to put on weight in their twenties: the target age for fashion advertising. Such weight control is a triumph, since the female body naturally comprises 26 per cent fat compared with 12 per cent for the male. Female sex hormones encourage fat storage, while male hormones enhance muscle-building. Young men in the higher income brackets in Britain eat 20 per cent more calories than those less well-off doing harder physical work. Nearly 30 per cent of young male professionals are overweight at 35. From their thirties onwards the proportion of fat women slowly increases, but not until the decade 55–64 do women – just – overtake men in the weight stakes. Right through their sixties and seventies more and more women put on extra weight, while the number of fat men declines. Nevertheless, the women outlive the men. In the United States, where immigration has produced a multi-ethnic mix, a review of those in the middle-income group – to avoid the poverty factor – showed that 4 per cent of fourth-generation Americans are too fat, compared with 92 per cent first- and second-generation Czechoslovakian Americans, 23 per cent Italian and 16 per cent Irish. Occupation has a twofold influence on figure: what is acceptable for the job and the effect of the work itself. Models, dancers, jockeys and aircrew are slim; cooks, barmen and bus-drivers may not be. Athletes may be abnormally low in fatty tissue but muscular in the competitive phase. They risk replacing much of the muscle with fat later.

Some authorities see obesity in the West as a major health hazard. This is open to question. What is beyond doubt is the misery suffered by the many who see themselves as greedy and despicable because of a minor excess over some mythical ideal.

What use is fat?

Fat is a vital fuel store, a reserve for the muscles when they cannot be supplied from current intake, for instance during a round of golf, a boxing bout or a marathon. Indirectly fat for the muscles safe-guards the sugar supply for the brain, which can run on nothing else. In women a further use for fat is to ensure nutrition for the growing fetus and for breast-feeding at a time when a mother might have difficulty in getting her own food. Fat also provides cushioning and comfort over bony points, and insulation.

It was probably two million years ago, when man first walked upright, that the layer of fat under the skin became differentiated between the sexes. Males require only half as much fat reserve as females, and from 5 years old girls already have twice as much fat as boys. Females have an all-over fat layer, plus a major reproductive reserve. This is stored conveniently in the pelvic and thigh regions. The breasts comprise mainly glandular tissue, and fat in this area, except in preparation for breast-feeding, is not an especially feminine characteristic. This is frustrating for middle-aged women who tend to 'spread' below the waist while their breasts shrink. It is equally annoying for older men, particularly if they drink heavily, to develop thickened fatty deposits in this area.

The pear shape – stalk up – is certainly feminine and indicates plentiful oestrogens at the time when the fat was laid down. It is alarming for teenage girls to find themselves becoming this shape because of their hormones and regardless of diet. By contrast, with their upsurge of male hormone, adolescent boys lose fat from the waist down, allowing untrammelled mobility. Their main increase is over the shoulders and the nape of the neck. Cortisol enhances a typically male distribution of fat in either sex, and from the age of about fifty women tend to lay down fat over the upper arms, shoulders and nape – the widow's hump.

Fat metabolism

Apart from brown fat, with its unique function, fat metabolism is under hormonal and nervous control. Thyroid, growth hormone and cortisol have an influence and there are special terminals in fat for insulin, sex hormones and the nervous system. The latter is the main regulator for the release of fat from storage, working in conjunction with the hormones. It is particularly difficult for a woman past the menopause, low in hormones, to get rid of abdominal fat. Men are less handicapped, as their sex hormones do not switch off so sharply. In the first 6 months of pregnancy hip and thigh fat reserves are increased without extra food. This hormonally mediated build-up is very efficient in some mothers, but its reversal at the end of pregnancy is less reliable. Breast-feeding may 'remind' the body of its changing needs, but most women who bottle-feed regain their figures as satisfactorily as the others. Family history is the key: in some families there is a hereditary tendency to put on more weight with each baby.

General metabolism

This means all the activity in the cells of the body, using fuel and oxygen for energy. It includes the mechanisms that either build up or run down fat stores, and comprises three types: basal metabolism, heat production and physical activity.

Basic metabolism concerns the energy used to keep vital bodily functions ticking over and accounts for 50–75 per cent of total energy expenditure. Fat people have a high metabolic rate – although they like to believe the opposite – because under the fat they have also larger-than-average muscles to move around with.

The basal metabolic rate comes under the control of the thyroid hormones, which slow it down if there is a weight loss. This accounts for the disheartening plateau that often occurs after about 2 weeks on a slimming regime.

Energy is used up in digesting and processing the food eaten but, especially after a big carbohydrate meal, some of the surplus energy derived from it is burned away as heat instead of being stored as fat. Some of the drugs used in high blood pressure block this reaction, and the person does not experience the normal warm glow after a good meal. Nicotine stimulates heat production. The weight gain that commonly accompanies giving up smoking is due partly to increased appetite, partly to decreased heat energy expenditure. Surges of exciting emotion, good or bad, also bring on surges in metabolic rate: noticeable from the quickened pulse.

Exercise has general beneficial effects, but apart from sports professionals, most people spend less than two hours a day exercizing. This amounts to 300–400 kcals over the basic value of around 1500 kcals for 24 hours.

Weight regulation

Most people seem to believe that deliberate control of food intake is normal and necessary to avoid getting fatter and fatter: that lifelong, iron-willed dietary restraint is the only way. Books on the subject abound, each setting out a different formula of restrictions, with some foods absolutely forbidden, others rationed. In fact, whether a person is slim, plump or 'perfect' his or her weight usually remains relatively stable, through automatic adjustments. It reverts without conscious effort to what it was before a bout of gastroenteritis, a lazy hotel holiday, or a period of slimming.

There are two important theories of weight regulation: fiscal and set-point. The former runs like an accounts sheet: food calories in, activity calories out. If they do not balance precisely weight goes up or down ... but this is absurdly simplistic. Even with a pocket calculator in constant use, it would be impossible to keep tabs. How many more calories are used if you hit a tennis ball hard rather than strategically, and what about running around the court? Secondly, calories are not constant. Ten calories of courgettes are not the same nutritionally as ten calories of cake. The label 'less than 50 calories' on low fat yoghourt is a good selling ploy: but deceptive. Yoghourt is more 'fattening' than lettuce to the same value. Thirdly the eater's current metabolic state is critical. If she has recently lost weight, through dieting or otherwise, she will more easily replenish her fuel stores than if her fat reserves are already full. This accounts for a frustrating situation: although in the ordinary way a fattish person's weight is quite stable, if she has managed to starve off a few pounds and then relaxes ever so slightly, her weight will shoot up in what seems a most unfair manner. During pregnancy there is increased efficiency in the body's use of food, with a weight gain of about 13 kg (29 lb), much more than the womb and fetus. This weight increase does not require 'eating for two'.

Set-point theory
This is a useful concept, although the term is inaccurate. It is not so much a point but a range with predetermined limits. Even these limits are flexible, varying over 24-hour and 12-month periods. People weigh more at 6 p.m. than 6 a.m., and more in the Autumn than the Spring. The set-point depends upon an internal criterion concerning the body's energy reserves, which include fat. Eating is not caused by a permanent greed, working blindly to make a person fat, but a sensitive response to the needs of the fuel stores for replenishment to their usual state. Energy is being used all the time at a changing rate, whereas food is taken in periodically. It is fortunate for survival that automatic mechanisms maintain reasonable reserves independently of thought and will. Fat people and others finding difficulty in drastically restricting their food intake often complain that they are out of control. In fact they have a conflict of controls. On the one hand is conscious willpower trying to limit intake; on the other the tireless physiological demands, working to defend the set level of fat store. Most people who lose a substantial amount of weight go back to their original size over weeks, months or years: through changes in appetite for amount

and type of food, and more subtle internal adjustments. What is needed is to alter the setting.

The set-range varies in its daily and yearly rhythm, according to age and development, and with sex. More immediate modifiers of the setting include the sensory aspect: constantly available, varied and palatable food push the setting up, particularly since most of us are genetically programmed to seek pleasure. Exercise, by contrast, lowers the set-point. Limiting intake does not alter the set-point, but those who persistently pit their will against the natural mechanism may ultimately disorganize the body's system of signals about its needs. Both the emotional and the thinking aspects of eating may become uncoupled from the routine feedback arrangements. The victim no longer knows how much to eat or what hunger feels like. Anxiety, depression or falling in love may affect the appetite either way, but not via the set-point machinery.

Appetite

Appetite is central to the three phases of eating: the pleasurable start, the enjoyment of continuing, and the satisfied switch-off. Frank hunger, from alerting signals that reserves are running low, is unusual in present circumstances, but a rise in insulin sharpens the desire to eat. The smell or sight of delicious food induces an anticipatory increase in insulin – and in appetite. Some fat people run on a higher-than-average insulin level all the time. It used to be thought that a rumbling tummy was an important stimulus to eating, but the feeling of emptiness is more relevant. Nourishing food is normally held in the stomach for an hour or two, but some people, including anorexics, retain the meal for many hours and feel bloated. In others the stomach empties rapidly and is always ready for a refill. The pleasurable feelings associated with the beginning of a meal are due to endorphins, self-made opiates which give a sense of well-being. For most people the endorphin concentration falls quickly as the meal progresses, but in a minority it remains high and they are prone to go on eating too long.

Appetite is enhanced by variety. Most people, even if they feel full after the first course, find that they still have room to enjoy cheese or dessert. Unlike alcoholics, who tend to stick to the same drink, 'food-aholics' often deliberately select as many different textures and flavours as possible. Allaesthesia is an interesting phenomenon: given a choice of sugar solutions most people prefer a stronger or weaker solution according to whether they have recently had something sweet, but some of those inclined to overeat show no such discrimination. Knowing when to stop eating is an important feature of appetite. Cholecystokinin, a hormone from the gut, decisively switches off the desire to eat.

It used to be thought that an eating centre and a satiety centre in the brain controlled appetite. In fact there are no such centres but concentrations of fibres carrying influential chemical messengers. Medicines and social drugs may affect appetite via these neuro-transmitters or messengers. They are also affected by psychological upsets. In general, medication that increases the amount of nor-adrenaline in the nervous system leads to a boost of appetite, especially for carbohydrates, with consequent weight gain. The time spent eating and the amount eaten both go up. Mild anxiety states and the early stage of the cheerful phase in manic depression release extra noradrenaline – and increase food intake. Some medi-cines lead to an increase in another neuro-transmitter, serotonin. Unlike noradrenaline this leads to a preference for protein and a slight reduction in appetite. Steroid medicines and natural cortisol greatly enhance carbohydrate appetite, and missing a meal also stimulates noradrenaline release and suppresses serotonin. This is one reason why a slimmer who has foregone breakfast may be impelled to buy a chocolate bar at the first shop. Stress induces noradrenaline and cortisol production, a rise in blood pressure, reduction in sugar – and a feeling of apprehension. A sweet carbo-hydrate snack reverses all these effects: a child who is upset should be given sweets and an irritable man fed.

Among women patients in particular, a common excuse for not taking medicines that have been prescribed is the fear that they may cause weight gain. Such effects are small, but medication tending to encourage appetite includes:

1 Benzodiazepines, such as Valium.
2 Phenothiazines, such as Largactil.
3 Antidepressants, such as Tryptizol.
4 Steroids, such as prednisolone.
5 Lithium.

Neuroleptics: These are used mainly for serious psychiatric illnesses like schizophrenia. They increase appetite and blood sugar and are apt to cause lethargy. Long-term schizophrenics are often mildly overweight.

Antidepressants, particularly the tricyclic group including amitriptyline and imipramine, tend to increase weight. Appetite improves and there is a predilection for sweet foods.

Lithium, used to treat manic-depressive illness, often induces a few pounds' weight gain.

Social drugs: Cannabis and alcohol both encourage weight gain. Cannabis increases appetite and brings on a relaxed, dreamy state with little activity. 'Beer belly' is well known, but any alcoholic drink can lead to an accumulation of fat in the liver and a general increase. Later, if the liver is damaged by alcohol, there is increased cortisol production with a bloated, red appearance. Finally, as the liver fails, the drinker becomes thin.

Chapter 12

Shapes in Fatness: Apples and Pears

There are many causes of fatness. Its effects vary, depending on the type. Because of pejorative attitudes towards fat people and their own shame about their shape, they long for a cause that is purely physical, no more their fault than pneumonia. A handful of rare hereditary and glandular disorders fill the bill: for a tiny minority only. For these people their fat is the least of their problems. In the hereditary group bones, muscles, brain and sexual development are all abnormal. In the 'glandular' group the thyroid gland has attracted the widest interest. Most fat people have a normal thyroid, but in those with an underactive thyroid there may be an insidious increase of weight by up to 10 per cent: say from 63 kg (10 st) to 69 kg (11 st). Tests will confirm the condition. Treatment is simple and weight returns to normal. Cushing's syndrome results from excess of cortisol, normally produced by the adrenal glands: it is readily diagnosed through blood tests. It can develop as a result of treatment with steroids. Fat accumulates over the collar-bones, the nape of the neck and the trunk generally, and the cheeks become round and red.

Effects of fat on the glandular system

While the endocrine glands are an occasional cause of fatness, cause and effect are not always easy to disentangle. Extra fat in itself can increase cortisol production, and produce an appearance like Cushing's syndrome. In fat girls the periods start abnormally early and are likely to be irregular. Fat men have low levels of male hormone, with reduced libido and even impotence. These abnormalities right themselves automatically when weight reverts to normal.

There are two types of fatness from eating more than the body needs: pear-shaped or gynoid, and apple-shaped or android.

Pear pattern

This comprises an exaggeration of the female shape, with a concentration of plumpness between waist and knees. The pear shape is ungainly, may be uncomfortable fitting into an aircraft seat, and causes wear and tear on the knees and feet, but there is little likelihood of a health disaster or early death – unlike the apple shape. Fat ladies are usually pears, and a few men: they are the lucky ones. Professor Vague, studying the shape of fat people for the past 40-odd years complains of the injustice to those, mainly men, who are no fatter than the pears but who carry their fat differently, and run considerable health risks. The lives of fat, pear-shaped women are not shortened, but the minority of women who develop the male pattern of fat also die like men – early.

Apple pattern

In this the waist is wider than the hips. Fat is concentrated on the upper trunk, with abdominal fat starting above the navel, and much of it packed beneath the muscles rather than just under the skin. Excess cortisol both leads to and is enhanced by this fat distribution: a vicious circle. The metabolic consequences may be disastrous. They include:

1 Raised blood pressure, predisposing to stroke and heart attack.
2 Extra fat in the blood, hyperlipidaemia, leading to:
3 Deposits of fat in the arteries, atherosclerosis, worsening the effects of high blood pressure.

4 Raised uric acid in the blood, predisposing to gout.
5 Raised insulin levels, interfering with sugar metabolism.

Diabetes mellitus, maturity onset type, commonly reveals itself after a fat person has reached and passed his or her maximum weight: the diabetes comes out when the metabolism is beginning to fail and the sufferer has lost 2–3 kg (4–6 lb) without trying.

Apple, unlike pear pattern fatness, increases the risk of heart and artery disease just as much as smoking, high blood cholesterol, or high blood pressure from separate causes. The reason for the ominous significance of fat concentrated above the navel lies mainly in the differences in fat metabolism according to its site. Fat on the bottom, lower abdomen, thighs and just under the skin generally, can only be mobilized slowly, and in the presence of the sex hormones, for possible use as fuel. This means that only a small quantity of fat gets into the blood at any one time. By contrast, fat inside the abdomen, under the muscular wall, is released rapidly through stimulation of the sympathetic nervous system: which in turn is galvanized into action by stress or excitement. The effect is a surge of free fatty acids into the bloodstream, flooding the liver with work, dealing with the liquid fat, and making fatty deposits in the blood vessels en route. Presumably because their lives are more eventful and they are more emotionally reactive, it is young men, 25–30, whose health is most likely to be harmed in android-type fatness. An additional factor is a difference between male and female muscles. Men have more so-called fast-twitch muscle fibres: these run, very efficiently, on glucose. Women have many slow-twitch fibres, which can gradually burn fat for fuel, less powerfully.

Exercise

The results of regular, moderate exercise on fat also vary with its position. Without concurrent dieting weight remains the same in both types, but in pears there is slight increase in the proportion of fat to muscle. Apple-shaped men and women, who are more muscular to start with, show an increase in lean tissue and lose some fat.

There are advantages from exercise for both types, however. In all cases there is a lowering of blood pressure, a reduction of excess insulin and better use of glucose, a reduction in uric acid in the blood and some fats, and the development of more slow-twitch muscle fibres.

Chapter 13

100 Ways the Family Can Help Someone to be Fat

Progressive, developmental fatness, which grows with the child, is likely to last into adulthood, and it depends very largely on the parents – or whoever feeds the child.

Babies

Extra-nutritious feeding cannot happen with breast-feeding. The baby simply will not take more than he requires of the sweet, watery fluid, but a bottle may contain a concentrated or thickened mixture. Surplus nourishment fills the fat cells and at this age their number increases: a reservoir ever-ready for replenishment, all the child's life.

Babies' crying is peculiarly disturbing. Anxious mothers are desperate to do something to quieten it and feeding is most often effective: acting like a stopper, even if the baby is cold or bored rather than hungry. A young couple living with in-laws may feel it essential to keep a baby quiet. On the other hand, an unhappy mother whose marital relationship is in conflict, and who is deriving no joy from motherhood, may stuff her baby with nourishment in the hope that he will sleep for most of the time and need minimal attention from her. Some mothers tend to go against ideal medical advice, from doctor or clinic, and change from breast to bottle and tend to use thickened feeds sooner than the baby needs: helping him to become plump. Feeds are often backed up by mini-bottles of sweet juice. Even a plain dummy teaches the baby an important lesson towards becoming and staying fat: that all comfort, all pleasure, comes in through the mouth and attempts at communicating other needs and feelings are fruitless. The answer will be oral anyway. Like the extra fat cells these concepts, once acquired, are durable.

When a baby becomes a toddler he can still be helped towards obesity, despite his natural proclivity for increasing crawling, climbing, walking, throwing. Little children readily develop a taste for such energy-rich, effort-free foods as chocolate biscuits – given the opportunity. They also readily get into the habit of eating or sucking something all of the time rather than mainly at meals. Another ploy for helping a child grow fat is to restrict his physical outlets: an early introduction to television provides passive sitting rather than romparounds and trips to the park. Living in a high-rise flat in the inner city makes it a major undertaking for a mother to arrange outdoor play for her young child. This is followed up later by restricting a schoolchild's going out to play or even to walk to school, because of the dangers.

Family influences on a child's eating

Grandparents can help their grandchildren to put on fat by showing their love regularly: with sweets, or money to buy them. They are often prone to praise a child – to his parents – as bonny, sturdy or well-built when in truth he is heavy and podgy. It is not surprising that parents, abetted by grandparents, frequently fail to recognize that their child is abnormally fat. In the same vein, even when, under doctor's guidance, a child has managed to slim down, his fond disbelieving mother may slyly re-feed him. In families where many members are 'big', and heavy eating may be the habit, it is easy for parents to regard their child's overweight as inevitable, instead of assessing the risk factors and taking avoiding action. It is disheartening for a child, particularly a daughter, to believe that she is doomed to fatness.

Only, youngest and especially precious children are at risk of being made fat. Belinda's parents were besotted by their beautiful baby, the reward for years of trying to procreate; Robin's parents nearly lost him from pneumonia in infancy. In each case the parents reacted by over-indulgence, including nutritional. It encourages a child to become fat if his parents are clearly delighted when he eats, and he is taught that it is 'good' to finish everything. Compliance and passivity are hallmarks of children who have allowed themselves to be coerced into becoming fat. Parents who have at any time in their lives suffered deprivation and hardship are likely to develop an almost superstitious insistence that their child should eat – and eat. This was noticeable among Jewish refugees from Hitler's Europe when they arrived in the USA: a generation of overfed children resulted, who felt guilty all their lives if they 'wasted' any food. Mothers are more closely involved than fathers with feeding, but some rich and successful men who see their children as possessions are interested in what they eat. One such father boasts of his 6-year-old son whose tastes are so sophisticated that his favourite dish is escargots. Dominic is affected somewhat similarly: unfortunately he demonstrated neither athletic prowess nor academic brilliance but his father was proud of the impressive quantities of food his son could consume. Dominic is obese.

A fatness-promoting family eating style may include hearty meals suitable to a long-past agricultural lifestyle on the one hand, or on the other may consist of an unstructured plethora of pizza, pasta and a varied range of pre-cooked meals and take-aways. Technological advance is almost all directed at saving physical effort, and calories. Aside from the obvious labour-saving devices in the home, it is calculated that a single telephone extension saves 70 miles of walking per annum, equivalent to 1–1.5 kg (2–3 lb) of fat. The constant availability of food in the home means that a child – or adult – who is fed-up, bored or lonely is likely to eat something, even if he is not hungry. The domestic refrigerator increases the range of what is on offer. It is significant that while from Monday to Friday 70 per cent of television advertisements for food concern high-calorie products, at weekends this rises to 85 per cent.

In families where there is discord between the parents, the child is often seen as some kind of compensation, and provider of affection in a bleak set-up. Neither parent can let the child develop his own independence but each becomes possessive, clinging and over-powering – and competes to indulge the child. Sometimes one partner recognizes a fat child's need to restrict his intake, but the other will more than make up for this. Mothers on their own may feed their children extra-generously, expressing their own need for nurturing. Most likely to become fat is a child whose sibling has died. He will be fed compulsively, as though that will ensure he stays alive, while his lifestyle is limited by his parents' fears. A different aspect of illness in the family arises when one child is chronically ill or handicapped, and absorbs so much of his parents' time and attention that the other child is barely noticed. In these circumstances, and others involving insecurity, anxiety and depression, the 'fit' child is liable to comfort himself by eating to fatness. Another type of parental management that drives an already vulnerable child further into obesity is continual criticism of his or her eating. Mrs Westcott was a small-boned thin woman married to a man built on generous lines: their daughter resembled him physically. Mrs Westcott lost no opportunity of pointing out Jennifer's ungainly size and plumpness, and her taste for all the wrong foods – for her own good, of course. The constant humiliation induced a defiant reaction rather than compliance. When her mother pointed out that pastries are fattening, Jennifer took three: regardless of the fact that she would be the main sufferer.

Meanings of food

It is during childhood, and from parents more than peers or teachers, that basic concepts are learned: including those concerning food. Food is a necessity and the older generations refer to 'keeping up one's strength' and promote various foods as 'good for you' as opposed to good or enjoyable to eat. Food often implies sharing life: parents in particular may see it as uniting the family. But the Sunday lunch ritual is losing favour in Britain with older children who prefer to have snacks with their own generation. Food is used for celebrating, and as a reward. It also may be withheld as a punishment, from political prisoners, and by parents who send recalcitrant children to bed without supper. Both these ways of using food give it especial value. Foods defined as treats are traditionally energy-rich: *boeuf-en-croûte*, sherry trifle, Christmas cake. Food may be a gift, between friends and lovers, most particularly within the family from mother, almost a part of herself. Woe betide the child or husband who 'turns his nose up' at the offering. Food can mean being cared for, looked after: witness the excessive pleasure caused to the usual provider if a child makes her a cup of tea.

Food may be regarded as a panacea: not only for peevish babies but for anyone suffering cold, pain, worry, fatigue, disappointment, sadness, shock – or hunger. Hot milk is the recognized specific for insomnia; no matter what distress or anxiety is keeping sleep at bay. It is maladaptive for a child to learn that, whatever is wrong, eating will alleviate it, rather than exploring the causes and discussing solutions. Most of those with eating disorders come from families in which communication is a disregarded skill. The Taggarts were this type. Mrs Taggart loved her son, all the more intensely when his pretty younger sister began to outstrip him academically and in popularity and became their father's pride and delight. Instead of discussing the situation with her husband and working out ways to raise Bobby's self-esteem, she favoured him silently by giving him the biggest portions and little extras when he came in from school. As he became fatter and unhappier she redoubled her efforts, until his only pleasure was eating and she was the main source of supply. At puberty Bobby began to have the normal interest in girls, but found himself out of the running, and with a burden of fat.

Adolescence

This is a period, starting at puberty, of profound change and upheaval, fundamentally involving relations within the family. The adolescent's major task is the establishment of his sexual and personal identity, reassessing parental views and values, discarding as necessary, and redirecting his loyalties towards his own generation. The price is the relinquishment of dependency: alarming for the individual and likely to be resisted by his parents. While his or her body is changing and his feelings towards life, himself and other people are in a state of flux, his appetite and eating may also run into chaos. Exuberant growth may take him by surprise. During the first half of this century the size and shape of adolescents in the West has altered. Boys of sixteen-plus average 4 cm (1.6 in) more in height, 4.5 kg (10 lb) extra weight; but girls, although taller by 1 cm (0.4 in) are lighter by 1.5 kg (3.2 lb) in the 16–19 age group. This sexual divergence implies that girls more than boys are likely to be struggling against nature to restrict their intake. The danger is of a reaction of overeating under stress or in the relaxation of fatigue.

The family's role is all-important in fostering the adolescent's self-esteem and independence. Criticism, intended as kindly advice, crushes the youngster's desperately frail confidence that he will be able to handle adult responsibilities. It may be tempting to remain – a little longer – immature, a good child, cared for and fed by mother: and fat. However an adolescent finds herself overweight, her – or his – sense of control will dwindle, and she is likely to withdraw socially. This may have a beneficial effect on study, gaining parents' and teachers' approbation. Another reinforcement to remaining over-plump, that applies only to girls, is an impression that their mothers would not welcome a slim, attractive, young rival. It can be a relief to opt out of sexual competition with contemporaries, with a morale-saving myth that a little slimming later will revolutionize the position.

The family can help ensure that a fat adolescent remains so: by exhortations to go out socially, when humiliation is certain; by advice of the obvious, to eat sensibly and exercise more; and by critical comparison with successful teenage friends. Fathers especially lower still further the social confidence of overweight adolescents by a noticeable lack of enthusiasm for their company, particularly with prestigious friends. A family in conflict is likely to produce a food addict or worse, a daughter tending to use food, a son to use drugs. Family tension added to adolescent anxieties is too much to bear unameliorated. Some less overtly conflictual parents cannot face a holiday together without the dilution of their teenage child's company. If the family holiday means food, drink, lazing in the sun and little activity, most members will return with added pounds, including the adolescent. Swimming, surfing, ski-ing or mountaineering in his own age-group will not have this effect.

Most parents of overweight adolescents are concerned. If this concern is basically derogatory it will not improve the teenager's tendency to eat too much and withdraw from activities with others. Equally it is counterproductive for parents to involve themselves with matters appropriate to a much younger child: homework, meals, clothes, late nights. This inhibits their adolescent's progress towards a mature, self-reliant attitude. If a daughter is dieting, whatever her mother does is likely to cause offence. Providing special low-calorie dishes for the dieter invokes jealousy of the others; reassuring her that a morsel of a favourite food 'can't do any harm this once' arouses fury. Help and advice may be sought but are received as interference.

Adult life

It is the marital partner or equivalent who has the most influence. Poor communication – of feelings, hopes and fears – propels a vulnerable partner towards some other form of relief. Food is always available and is not immediately detectable like alcohol, drugs or an affair. If a husband is made redundant or a wife has a miscarriage support is more effective than food. Support is measured in personal time, with a readiness to listen, and then some shared distractions. Douglas's wife felt lost when her sister died unexpectedly. Her husband hit on the time-saving (for him) manoeuvre of buying her a dog for comfort and companionship. Both she and the animal became fat on chocolate, and her grief was unresolved.

Pregnancy is a period when a woman lays down fat physio-logically. This may never be lost, either because of constitutional tendencies or from psychological factors. A husband who appreci-ates his wife as a good mother rather than a desired lover helps her to matronliness. A woman who feels unattractive may relax all efforts to keep up her self-pride. She may never change clothes, seldom open a book, avoid exercise and compensate for a feeling of emptiness by passive sensual activities such as visits to the hairdresser or snacking. On the other hand, it has been demonstrated that if a husband often criticizes his wife's figure or food intake she is likely to get fatter in defiance or despair.

Similarly with men of 40-plus: Mrs W., having borne her two children, was no longer interested in intercourse, and made this clear. She was, however, a cordon bleu cook and did not withhold this skill. Tom W. took to girlie magazines, masturbation and sumptuous meals. He is now obese in the apple shape and awaits bypass surgery. His wife, even fatter but in the pear mode, is unscathed. Husbands and wives can help each other achieve and maintain a high level of fatty tissue by focusing their joint interests on eating out, drinks with friends, luxury hotel holidays – and no distractions like music, the theatre, sport or wild-life. Sexual activity becomes less appealing, less satisfactory, less casy: particularly with each other.

Chapter 14

Methods for Making and Keeping Yourself Fat

Whatever the motivation, the basic manoeuvre for putting on weight is persistently to take in more nourishment than is used. However, it is inaccurate and unkind to say that fat is simply due to overeating. Among middle-aged men in the Netherlands the 25 per cent with the highest weights were found to consume 300–400 kcal less, daily, than those with the lowest weights. Presumably the fatter men who ate less had sedentary work and access to the full range of modern electronic and mechanical gadgets. In Glasgow a comparison of adolescents in 1964 and 1971 showed that the later group ate less than the earlier, but had more body fat. The explanation must lie in the greater use of parents' cars and an increase in passive entertainment. Similarly, while the prevalence of overweight in the USA has increased during this century, 5 per cent less energy per person is eaten. A technological culture means a steadily declining need for nourishment. Far from eating more from the ever-widening choice, the town-dweller today must deliberately cut down his intake to keep in step with his reduced energy requirement – or get fat.

Environmental changes are beyond individual control, but there are a number of conscious choices that will influence fatness.

Choice of food

Energy-dense foods, such as fish fried in batter, sausage rolls, cream éclairs, sweets and confectionery take little or no preparation and do not fill the stomach. Developing a taste for these foods is easy and probably happens early in life. Retraining established preferences is often strongly resisted. The person on the path to obesity will say with an air of finality: 'But I've never liked lettuce'. While some of those who want to control their weight carefully eschew potatoes, rice and pasta, in themselves low-density nutrients, they readily eat cheese – a concentrate of saturated fats. Similarly, they will accept boring bread and low-fat margarine: far more calorific than bread with jam or honey. Fats, weight for weight, provide more than twice as much energy as carbohydrate or protein and can be taken in almost imperceptibly with other foods. Sclafani's diet, really effective in fattening rats and humans, includes a variety of easily absorbed high-density foods: cake, chocolate, sandwiches, crisps, biscuits. Alcoholic drinks are a powerful adjunct.

Apart from the type of food, quantity is clearly of crucial importance. There are several ways of packing it in.

Nibbling

This comprises almost non-stop, day-long eating, in small doses: for instance a packet of twenty biscuits in an hour-and-a-half. Chefs and housewives are prone to tasting and tidying up which never produce the sensation of being uncomfortably full – and can continue. Calorie for calorie less fat is laid down by nibblers than gorgers, because they also build up muscle.

Unconscious eating

This is a curious mental phenomenon in which a person eats extra food unobserved, denies having eaten it, and seems unable to remember how it happened. Cooks' sampling often arises in this way, but larger amounts of food can also 'disappear'. Some quite fat people have this quirk and seem genuinely puzzled over where the food has gone.

Addictive eating

Some personalities have a propensity for becoming dependent on a habit: cigarettes, alcohol, gambling – or food, especially the kinds enjoyed in childhood. These include sweets, cakes, biscuits, breakfast cereals, ice-cream and bread and jam. The habit may develop during periods of loneliness or anxiety, but with repetition it imperceptibly gets a grip. The victim, like other junkies, feels increasingly restless, irritable and preoccupied with thoughts of food, within 2 or 3 hours of the last 'fix'. Concentration is impaired and the patient can feel ill and headachey. Neither friendship, sex nor figure matter and there is no compunction about taking someone else's food from a shared refrigerator or finishing off the office biscuits. Women are more often affected than men, but not exclusively. While the former are continually exposed to the temptations of food, the latter more naturally turn to alcohol. This can lead to a beer belly or its equivalent, but many established, serious drinkers eat and absorb too little nourishment to get fat.

Bingeing

This is often part of a seesaw. A girl or young woman – nearly always – who tends to put on more weight than is currently fashionable may live in a chronic state of struggling for control. She never enjoys a guilt-free meal, but is constantly trying to eat less than her appetite demands. She may miss meals, most often breakfast. The backlash occurs when she is tired, angry or has had a drink or tranquillizer. When the controls are relaxed she will allow herself to eat. Once started she will not stop until she has used up all that is available, with a bias towards what the addictive eater prefers. Sometimes she will deliberately set out to buy the food for a binge, choosing a variety of textures and flavours, but nothing that requires long preparation. On some occasions the binger stops because she can physically manage no more and feels full to the point of illness. The binger eats on through the initial discomfort, past satiation. If she lies down she is likely to fall asleep. The signs of devastation when she wakes up fill her with shame and guilt and she gets right back into the under-eating mode of the cycle. If she binges fairly frequently she will become fat, unless she puts into operation the patterns of bulimia nervosa and attempts to get rid of the food by self-induced vomiting or large doses of laxatives. Only the first of these methods is effective.

Night eating

This is a variant of bingeing, less extreme in quantity. It seldom affects young adolescents, but more often young women who are discontented in marriage or have unsatisfactory boyfriends, and sense a lack of affection. Starving all day and having a huge evening meal is commonplace among slimmers. Night-eating is somewhat different. It entails waking from sleep, getting up and creeping to the kitchen. It has some resemblance to unconscious eating as the woman feels as though she is eating in a dream, alone and unseen.

Reactive overeating

Bingeing and night-eating comprise one type of reactive overeating – eating excessively in reaction to chronic over-control. The other type is eating overmuch either in bouts or steadily at all meals, as a response to relieve depression, anxiety, interpersonal problems or the tension of boredom. This way of trying to deal with dysphoric emotions has usually been learned in childhood. With help and support it may be exchanged for reliance on human contact. Kummerspeck, 'the fat of sorrow', was so named in relation to war widows. An intolerable situation such as having an alcoholic spouse or a senile relative to look after can produce the same consequence – of tippling biscuits or sherry or both, and giving oneself compensatory food treats. Stress, either physical such as cold or fatigue, or psychological, either chronic or short-lived may impair the appetite of some people. But those already plump respond by eating more. Major changes – in home, job or family, whether for better or worse – engender stress. For example, a holiday is an episode intended to be beneficial but which involves the stress of strange surroundings, disrupted routine and not least, close continuous contact with nearest and dearest.

External cue responses

Most people eat according to a rhythm of appetite and timing interwoven with physiological prompting on the type of food and amount, i.e. internal cues. Others, some of whom are overweight, eat according to external cues, overriding their own bodily information. If they are offered food they accept and finish it all: a sequel of early 'clean plates' training. A solid meal is eaten at lunchtime or dinner, regardless of weather or activity. At a hotel or restaurant all that is included in the price is consumed. With friends and relatives, the potentially fat person responds to what his hostess seems to want, but even at an eating session where there is no hostess, he will eat more if more is provided. At a recent food fair in London huge baskets of sweetmeats were displayed for children accompanying their parents. In fact, the supplies were severely depleted by adults, already plump, helping themselves to handfuls. The sight of a baker's, a fast-food bar, or an inn will remind the external responder to eat, and the television advertisements also jump out at this type. A celebration or a distress, or merely seeing a friend is a signal to eat and drink. However, a readiness to respond to external rather than internal food cues need not be associated with overeating. For this to occur it must be coupled with ignoring the signals to stop eating. While they respond positively to the attractive appearance and smell of food, and its palatability, fat external responders are put off more and eat less than others if there is something wrong with the food.

Eating to communicate

Patients with anorexia nervosa convey, in disguised form, by their refusal to eat, particular forms of adolescent distress. The overweight too may eat to communicate feelings they cannot or dare not express in words. The message, often inaccurate, may be that they do not care about or are afraid of being sexually attractive; that they are big and strong, rejecting femininity; that they are warm and loving and want to share; that they are starving emotionally; that they wish they were pregnant; or that they are angry and hostile.

Avoiding activity

Exercise accounts for 20–30 per cent of energy expenditure. Those in very active occupations usually carry less fat than the average. A lumberjack can burn 5000 kcals a day fuelling his muscles. A fat man in a sedentary job may not be able to use up 2000 – and adds to his body stores. Forced inactivity from accident, handicap or some chronic illness calls for a thoughtful cutback in energy intake or weight will increase. In general fat people exercise less than normal.

Plump teenage girls float rather than swim when they bathe, and when they play tennis move around the court only 23 per cent of the time, compared with 77 per cent as norm. It is even more probable that the person who is to become fat will find that he or she is too busy for sport – except watching at Wimbledon, Lords or Wembley – and the least likely to be a keen or even dutiful gardener or engage in vigorous housework. Thin, wiry women spring-clean. Fat men walk less than others, but for fat women compared with average, the disparity is even more marked: 2 miles a day instead of 5. Interestingly, introducing a regular programme of exercise does not increase food intake in the long term, and appetite may even decline slightly. The hypothesis that obesity may be a disease of inactivity seems at least plausible.

Psychological aspects

Low self-esteem and hatred of one's own body make it easier to stuff it with rubbishy snacks and oddments, denying it well-balanced, properly spaced meals and a programme of physical activity. Adolescents are particularly likely to be harshly self-critical, feeling that personal failure and fatness are overtaking them. For those adolescents or adults who are in fact plump, ugly shapeless garments, or worse, worn-out relics of an earlier, slimmer phase stretched hideously over the swollen body reinforce a conviction of worthlessness. No new clothes are to be bought until an impracticable weight loss has been achieved.

Involutional despair: The effect of the menopause, male or female, is a blow to *amour-propre*. A woman has the dismal knowledge that her reproductive powers are spent, but not her husband's. A man finds the sexual act slower to start and to finish, and occasionally it fails completely and frighteningly. Even well-maintained bodies of a half-century plus show signs of wear and tear, with loss of muscle tone, and bulk made up to with extra fat, often more than enough to maintain the same weight. The skin, hair and bodily decline and the tendency to become fatter and flabbier can make the individual feel that he or she is no longer worth bothering about. To underline the point, there are likely to be adolescent offspring around, radiating sexuality, bloom and vigour. No wonder that middle-aged parents tend to give up self-care and settle for the simple pleasures of expense-account lunches, whisky and wine as a daily habit, not a treat. Fatness follows.

Chapter 15

Why Not Stay Fat?

Losing weight is difficult but commonplace. Keeping it off is a hundred times more difficult, and rare. Hilde Bruch, the guru of eating problems, suggests that ineffectuality is the hallmark of personality in fat people: but they have no single recognizable personality type. All sorts can have weight problems, including innumerable dynamic, successful action men and women. Aside from the group, 90 per cent female, of near-average weight who are obsessed with kilograms and kilojoules and thoroughly dissatisfied with their bodies, there are a huge number, somewhat overweight according to fashion, apparently trying to reduce. Why do they so seldom succeed for long?

There are hurdles at every stage for those who want to be thinner. Many Westerners, unlike Asians, are conditioned towards enjoyment, for which eating is an ever-available facility. It is tempting to postpone dieting until tomorrow, or after Christmas. The start of an exercise programme is even more frequently delayed because of the embarrassment of being seen in a leotard or swimsuit, or – for a man especially – performing abysmally. During the first 10 days of dieting the slimmer is liable to feel cold, tired, irritable, headachey and unable to concentrate: while certain relief is forbidden. The early drop-out rate is understandably high, with less than half of those who have made a commitment or contract turning up even for one in six of the meetings or appointments they have arranged. Slips on a dieting programme are universal, but they make some people feel that they are cheats as well as fat. They are ashamed to present themselves, and decide to wait until they have some success to show. Perhaps.

If the dieter does not give up at this stage, further adverse effects of the restrictions make themselves felt, including disturbed sleep and daytime restlessness. Characteristically the longer-term dieter feels unfairly deprived and resentful. Aggressive feelings strain relationships at home and work. Gradually the unpalatable insight emerges that it is likely to take months of effort to establish an acceptable weight: one at which ordinary clothes stores will stock your size. Even then there is no let-up. The price of staying slender – continued dieting – evokes great bitterness since others who have always been slim can apparently eat at will and much more than the slimmer. To keep down a recently reduced weight requires indefinitely prolonged restraint. This may produce specific problems. Low food intake brings on the starvation reaction: a reduced metabolic rate to conserve energy. Slowed-down metabolism is depressing to mood and vitality. Periods may stop. Eating enough to restore the metabolism to normal may also be enough to cause weight gain: a no-win situation.

This can be the beginning of the dreaded 'rhythm method of girth control', comprising alternating periods of harsh, unrealistic dieting and of relaxation to the level of indulgence. Weight is endlessly lost and regained, resulting in chronic failure, low confidence, bad eating habits and neither hope nor insight.

Young adults and women in particular often believe that achieving a weight similar to their peers' will bring about all they envy in other people: a more productive, happier lifestyle with success in every area. In fact, weight loss is often a disappointment. Part-way through, say after the first 2 kg (5 lb), the visible result may be negligible and others may still make scathing comments. It is disillusioning to the nth degree to struggle to the target and find that the quality of life does not improve. New snags may appear. A substantial weight loss alters a person's view of herself, and also that of other people. Children may be thrown by their mother's changed appearance. A man who felt at ease with a comfortably cushioned mate may find, like the author Anthony Burgess, that it is less enjoyable going to bed with someone like a bicycle. Admiration for a successful slimmer's willpower and fortitude does not increase other people's liking for her, and so does little to lift her self-esteem. On the other hand it can be downright alarming for a woman who has been accustomed to non-specific friendliness from both sexes to find that men are showing a different, expectant interest.

The advantages of plumpness can easily outweigh those of chronic dieting. The sharp edges of depression and anxiety are softened by eating, and fat people rarely commit suicide. Size confers a sense of presence and importance. The swinging stride of a fat woman or big man exudes confidence. Other women welcome the company of someone fatter than they are: it makes them feel slim. For those who have been overweight from childhood there is a feeling of security in maintaining the status quo. Adolescents fearful of facing the responsibilities of adulthood find that eating too much binds them in a child-like way to mother; advance into maturity is slowed. Sexuality may be put into abeyance. Fantasies about sexual adventures can flourish in adult or adolescent, so long as the perception of excess fat can be used to ward off reality. At a practical level, for the middle aged who so often run into weight gain, plumpness protects the skin from wrinkling, the neck from becoming scrawny and the breasts from atrophy. Most people of 40-plus who have recently lost weight, of either sex, look haggard in the face, withered in the limbs and oddly corrugated over the abdomen. If swimming gear is cruelly revealing for those with bulges, it is no better for the formerly fat.

There is an undoubted biological basis for bodily form, which it is sensible to accept, particularly if a parent is the same shape. For some people, regardless of heredity, becoming fat is the best adjustment they can manage to cope with their neurotic sufferings. These may include moodiness, dependency, low self-opinion, anxiety or a pervading sense of unimportance and loneliness. To remove eating as a resource leaves such sensitive people unprotected.

Overweight can be used as an excuse to avoid alarming social situations. Indeed, fat girls, because they pass up so many invitations and activities, often do well academically. Boys who are plump do not use their time so constructively. Some families and marriage partners communicate through food. This may not be the best way but it is better than emotional silence through dieting. Sharing food can convey sharing life, loving, looking after, rewarding, commiserating, celebrating, an indication of success, or a gift: according to context.

There are plenty of people undoubtedly fatter than fashion approves who are socially and personally well adjusted. They accept themselves and are accepted. No change is necessary. There are others, outwardly similar, who are constantly striving to alter their shape, and constantly worrying. They often eat in secret but refuse dishes prepared by others. While extra fat need not require a remedy, obsessive concern about shape certainly does.

Chapter 16

Treatments Tried and Discarded

There is no shortage of treatments for unwanted fat. Some people lose weight by one or another method, but for most of them the benefit is passing, since nothing else in their lives has changed. While most treatments are ineffectual in the long term, a few are downright dangerous, but most people who feel too fat want to know about them all.

Formal weight-reducing regimens

The cheapest ploy is to buy a book on slimming: new ones come out constantly. Most of them comprise recipes and menus – compulsive reading for those preoccupied with food. Some of the diets are gimmicky or based on false premises: Eat Fat and Grow Slim, The Scarsdale, Beverley Hills, F-Plan and Rotation Diets respectively. The calorie tables incorporated in these books can be deceptive: the poor digestibility of some high-density foods such as plum cake and Brazil nuts means that they actually provide less nutrition than low-density pasta. Even with books following sound nutritional principles, most people fail to get off and keep off their unwanted pounds. No-one can resist tinkering with the prescribed menus, and making exceptions of Sundays, Saturdays . . .

Groups and individual counselling on diet

Diet combined with self-help or commercial groups or individual counselling sessions is also likely to fail after the course has finished, if not before. There are drop-outs at every stage from outset to follow-up, and the functional drop-outs who turn up for meetings but do not comply with the advice. The long-established Weight Watchers organization includes a reward system in its package: weekly meetings and weigh-ins for which the individual must pay, with public praise for satisfactory loss, and a gift if it is substantial. Unfortunately most studies of slimmers who lost weight up to 10 years previously show hardly any still below their original overweight. This is not surprising since most will have returned to the same conditions in which they initially put on weight.

Men are likely to take up squash or other exercise to combat fat, but this alone is ineffective. Used in conjunction with diet it helps to preserve muscle and tone up the body. Genuinely fat women avoid exercise, but those already slim eagerly do aerobics.

Very low calorie (liquid) diets

These drastic artificial diets, which in no way resemble normal meals, provide 300–500 kcal daily. They acquired a sinister reputation in the late 1970s when a number of patients using low-quality liquid protein supplements died: their hearts stopped. Since then the formulae have been modified and there are several safer diets available. One of the best-known and most-researched is the Cambridge Diet. Even this may upset the digestive system in various ways, and periods on the diet must be interspersed with others on real food. As with all strict régimes, only 24 per cent of those who start actually complete the course and less than one in ten achieves the weight loss planned, even temporarily. The leading nutritionist, J.S. Garrow, considers very low calorie diets dangerous and unnecessary. Those who weigh more than the average invariably have a rate of energy-expenditure such that an 800–1000-calorie diet will cause weight loss without undue loss of muscle tissue which would in turn slow down the metabolism. Loss of muscle may never be fully restored by refeeding, as evidenced by prisoners-of-war and severe anorexics.

Drugs

There is a natural propensity for those with eating problems to want to take something by mouth as a cure. Slimmers beg for a magic tablet 'just to give me a start'. Most of the slimming drugs are nerve stimulants, acting like amphetamines or 'Speed'. The best known are diethylpropion, mazindol and phentermine (Tenuate, Apisate, Teronac, Duromine) – all are habit-forming, ineffectual in the long term and with a risk of physical and mental side-effects. These include headache, insomnia, irritability and tremor – and more seriously high blood pressure and paranoid psychosis. Fenfluramine (Ponderax) is an exception. It is not stimulating but helps the slimmer to stop more easily at the end of a meal. Some people develop a depression when they stop taking fenfluramine.

Filler-pills of bran, cellulose or dried seaweed swell in the stomach but do not satisfy the appetite. They may act as mild laxatives but have no other value. Chemical purges and diuretics require increasing doses and are harmful. They remove important chemicals and fluid from the body temporarily but have practically no effect on the fat stores or absorption of food. Thyroid hormones are usually ineffective since appetite increases to keep pace with the extra amount of hormone. Large doses are dangerous to the heart. A number of other drugs have been tried, for instance dinitrophenol, cholecystokinin, aspirin, ephedrine, methylxanthine, salbutamol, naltrexone, phenylpropanolamine, and nicotine. All of these are frequently being rediscovered and hailed as a 'breakthrough' in the popular press: all are dangerous to the point of disaster if taken in a dosage necessary to affect appetite or weight.

Mechanical methods

The gastric balloon is blown up inside the stomach: the major side-effect is intestinal obstruction.

Nylon girdle: Most people cannot resist cutting their unstretchable belt off as it becomes constricting.

Jaw-wiring: Apart from the anxiety of having to keep wire-cutters and pliers always at hand in case of choking, this method is ineffective in that many nourishing foods can be liquidized. Even with weight loss, it rapidly returns when the wires are off.

Surgery

Liposuction, a method of drawing off some of the abdominal fat in its natural liquid state, produces an oddly lumpy body as the fat reforms in patches.

Intestinal bypass was fashionable in the late 1970s, but the high risk of complications, some fatal, has led to its abandonment.

Operations on the stomach are still in the experimental stage, and further 'rescue' surgery is often needed.

Despite having braved the dangers of anaesthetic and major surgery – considerable in the overweight – some patients actually increase their fat reserves after these procedures. They choose soft nourishing foods and drinks. The compulsion to eat is not dealt with by surgery.

Since surgical, chemical, mechanical and artificial feeding methods of weight reduction are shot through with snags, a psychological approach may seem attractive.

Hypnosis: This is a favourite hope for neurotics, including some would-be slimmers, seeking a no-effort magical cure. While it is often useful for smokers it is useless in compulsive eaters or the slightly plump. No one can be programmed to believe that any or all food is harmful.

Behavioural psychotherapy is based on the principle of reward for good behaviour: difficult in an adult. Of course it is counterproductive to use a favourite food or drink as reinforcement for losing some weight. Praise or money is dull, while activity rewards – allowing the slimmer to do something he chooses – is often disappointing because nothing worthwhile seems feasible at the wrong weight. It might seem logical to combine behavioural treatment with fenfluramine, but the combination is even less effective than either treatment alone.

Feminism: Susie Orbach's approach really only applies to women.

Her first book, *Fat is a Feminist Issue*, was balm to the female soul, offering renewed self-respect. There is the reassurance that when women weigh more than they want, the fault is not in themselves. Far from being greedy, such women give too much and then – sadly – try to fill their own emptiness with food. Ms Orbach suggests that women should provide generously for their own needs and desires, including enjoyable food, in the hope that in a situation of plenty they may choose to say No. The girl or woman who feels fat is invited to visualize social scenes in which she is both thin and fat, and to develop a sense of her essential self. Group support from other women is felt to be important. This approach appeals to some women.

Chapter 17

Managing Life and Fat

Anyone can feel miserably fat, but it is more likely to be a female. Women have to pay for their partial access to male privilege by conflicting personal demands. They must have lean, designer bodies to be taken seriously as lawyers, stockbrokers, scientists, and something else to be lovable. A woman who feels fatter than perfection sees herself as inferior and hates her body. Her mind is focussed on a few pounds. Since everyone knows the connection between eating and fat, by the time she seeks help she will already have tried and failed to cut down. Most smokers say that they would love to stop – while making sure that their supplies do not get low. Similarly many of those claiming to be desperate to lose weight show nil motivation. Just as substantial and unfashionable size may be perfectly stable, so may the person's private acceptance of it. The refrain about wanting to reduce serves to ward off criticism and unwanted advice. This situation deserves recognition – and respect.

When there is a real desire to be different, and the individual believes her shape is the main fault, the first step is practical: comparing her weight-for-height with the average. Less than 10 per cent over the odds is negligible. Self-denigratory distress in these circumstances means that there must be a major cause hidden behind the front about being fat. At the opposite extreme are those, mainly men, with a fat load causing medical and family concern who brush aside any mention of a problem. This leaves a majority with mild to moderate surplus, and often disproportionately upset about it. Children may be very unhappy, particularly at school, but their weight problems are the parents' responsibility. Plumpness that develops in childhood becomes so much a part of the individual, distorting his personality and his physical appearance, that change in adulthood is almost impossible. Everything depends upon the parents, who need all possible help, and probably need to alter their own attitudes. An all-out effort to deal with a child's overweight before he is through adolescence is mandatory. A total family operation is required affecting not only eating habits but a major reorientation of shared interests and activities. Active involvement in sport, music, wildlife, politics – anything other than eating, drinking and watching the TV – is needed to distract attention from food. The fat child's enthusiasm must be aroused, his company and opinions appreciated and his successes praised. What adults do always seems attractive: it must also be healthy. Nagging criticism whether directly about eating or other deficiencies is counter-productive. A child who is shamed will eat for comfort or in defiance. Only the very best of parents will be able to turn their own lives upside down for the sake of their child.

Adolescents

Fat teenage boys are usually suffering from a surfeit or deprivation of mothering. Either way, it is their fathers and ultimately their own generation who can help them gain the confidence to face the adult world without the cover of being podgy. Similar ploys to those needed by younger children should be applied, but the mother's nurturing role is now outdated. Bribery to get a son started on some out-of-home pastime is money well spent.

Adolescent girls have a built-in difficulty in facing sexual maturity. Physiological changes make them fatter in a sensitive area, while at the same time raised oestrogen levels set off the sexual chemistry. This provokes a new kind of interest from boys and the girl herself has disturbing feelings. All this is frightening, but it is her bodily shape of which the adolescent girl is most acutely aware. It may be slightly reassuring to understand that the changes are normal and natural, but it may seem safer to let the unaccustomed female outline become blurred with extra fat, while eating is calming in itself. The snag is the damage to self-opinion from comparison with thinner, more confident contemporaries. Discrimination against the plump is present even in childhood. It increases dramatically among adolescents and the adults whom they meet. If either of her parents is big, the girl feels doomed, and if she has a slim, elegant mother she feels inadequate. Of course the girl needs to lose a few pounds, by her own efforts under her own control. Help, advice or encouragement from the family is not useful. Independence from mother – nothing to do with affection – is urgent, and practice in arguing down both parents is a step towards effective young adulthood. Leaving home emotionally and for real is of major benefit to self-opinion and to figure, without coming back too often for those old-fashioned, sit-down family Sunday lunches.

Men

Both young adults and middle aged may slip unawares into getting out of shape. A thirst for lager or wine with a fall-off of time spent on active sport can affect the young. Marriage may slow a man down to the pace of his youngest child, while his wife wants his company at home and may try to give him too much of all his favourite foods. It takes as much tact and determination to escape from loving, married domesticity as to get free from a loving, nurturing mother. Of course it is not all or nothing, but to avoid becoming tame and plump, most men need time and energetic sport with other males, as well as home time. By middle age most of the physical effort of work will have been transformed by promotion into shuffling papers, assisted by a secretary. The workaholic may revel in a 16-hour working day, with travel interspersed, but the harder he works the more time he spends sitting – in Concorde, in his Porsche, on the shuttle, in a boardroom. His sex life may be in jeopardy if he is too tired and frankly bored with what is available. Food may be the one sensual outlet that never fails. When a man has become, without doubt, overweight, the likelihood is that someone else will worry first. His wife may tell him that he must not eat or drink anything that he likes. She immediately puts herself in the nanny role, with her husband as the naughty child who will delight in outwitting her.

The doctor may try to focus anxiety on his patient's heart and blood pressure, joints or potential diabetes, particularly if such disorders run in the family, or serum cholesterol levels are high. Neither men nor women are likely to act on their doctors' warnings by altering their lifestyle – except when their career is at risk. A man who is afraid he may not be able to work is likely to react energetically, recklessly, by plunging into squash, jogging, mowing the lawn. A steady increase in mild exercise with a sharp reduction in gourmand-type meals and wines is safer, duller and more effective. If male aggression can be geared to beating a weight problem the battle is as good as won, but the man who cuts down to please someone else is programmed to fail.

Women

Young women, young mothers and the menopausal-plus – all are haunted by the spectre of themselves as fat. A woman's appearance determines how she is received socially, sexually, academically and in employment – from the first instant. Shape is the most influential feature, obvious from a distance, at any angle. Holiday wear hides nothing, hence the annual panic from late March to get into perfect trim for maximal exposure on the beaches. Those with more than 3 lb (1.5 kg) between them and model status may despair, while for the over-50s there is the constant sight of Joan Collins on TV to bring on feelings of inadequacy. Every woman worried about her weight is a unique individual but there are broad areas in common. The disorder urgently requiring relief is obsessive self-dissatisfaction based on a single aspect. It is easier for a woman to brood over her shortcomings than to celebrate her assets and achievements. Time should be spent on discussing how to enhance and make the best use of her positive traits: of character and personality, skills and knowledge, imagination and creativity and environmental advantages in say home, family, friends or finances. One likeable physical detail should be included. Weight falls into perspective.

A multi-faceted improvement and development programme must be planned on each person's positive qualities – nothing of value derives from the negative. Change and enrichment are the objectives, and should include new, constructive leisure activities, new learning, fresh adventure, and greater interaction with others. A figure-improving component can be included when the rest of the plan is in place, and the possibilities of success or shortfall do not all rest on diet. An absolute maximum for weight loss must be agreed at 6 lb (2.5 kg); any further weight adjustment must be delayed for at least a month. At that time general progress is assessed and an updated programme launched, if necessary. The method for weight adjustment involves daily exercise and fresh air for at least half-an-hour, and three compulsory meals daily with drinks between. A low-fat diet is far more effective than low carbohydrate, and such fillers as potatoes, rice, (non-egg) pasta and bread without spread can be eaten freely so long as they are not cooked with fat. This makes it easier not to feel hungry, and not to make others feel uncomfortable by eating like a rabbit. After 1 month or 6 lbs (2.5 kg) loss, whichever is the sooner, the slimmer can relax slightly, to maintain her weight at its new level, until the next programme is instituted.

Somewhat separately from the general improvement plan, a simultaneous advance should be made towards developing a happier outlook. The main plank for this is increased interaction with other people outside the family, sharing with them personal interests, thoughts and feelings rather than talking on impersonal subjects. Constructive activities aside from work – music, art, politics, sport, photography – are more rewarding than the purely social. Nevertheless, the most successful people in their casual and closer relationships are those who, shy or not, behave in an extrovert way: making contact with and interested in others. The neurotic who shrinks away because of her shape and avoids conversation brings about what she fears: she remains outside any group.

Allowing oneself to eat or drink more than is strictly sensible is natural and understandable, when it is so easy, relaxing and frankly enjoyable. Most people who are plumper than they would like, or even definitely overweight, are perfectly normal psychologically. It is not surprising or unreasonable that they are not content about it, perhaps unhappy or anxious about their image. If they can set themselves and achieve other objectives than often unrealistic ambitions for a sylph-like shape, and their general sense of well-being and competence rises, weight may become less preoccupyingly important.

Some people put on excessive fat in the context of a psychological illness: tension state, depression, bereavement reaction or one of the major psychoses. Treatment for the illness has total priority in these cases; the weight problem may subside later anyway. When it is urgently necessary to reduce weight, for instance before surgery, this is probably best managed in hospital. When there is an important but not critical medical indication to lose weight, twice weekly supervision, discussion and encouragement keeps the momentum going and offers the best chance of improvement.

While a balanced attitude with a dash of realism is essential to lasting weight change, some of the psychological manoeuvres outlined in Chapter 16 may be helpful – and no change at all occurs without dieting.

Further Reading

Bruch, Hilde, *The Golden Cage: The Enigma of Anorexia Nervosa*, Open Books Publishing Ltd, London, 1978

Brumberg, J., *Fasting Girls. The Emergence of Anorexia Nervosa as a Modern Disease*, Harvard University Press, Massachusetts, 1988

Chernin, K., *The Hungry Self. Women, Eating and Identity*, Virago Press Ltd, London, 1986

Conley, R., *The Complete Hip and Thigh Diet*, Arrow Books, London, 1989

Dally, P., Gomez, J. and Isaacs, A., *Anorexia Nervosa*, William Heinemann Medical Books Ltd, London, 1979

Garrow, J.S., *Treat Obesity Seriously*, Churchill Livingstone, London, 1981

MacLeod, S., *The Art of Starvation*, Virago Press, London, 1981

Minuchin, Salvador, *Families and Family Therapy*, Harvard University Press, Cambridge, Massachusetts, 1974

Orbach, S., *Fat is a Feminist Issue*, 2nd edn., Arrow Books, London, 1988

Selvini, Mara P., *Self-starvation: From the Intrapsychic to the Transpersonal Approach to Anorexia Nervosa*, Chaucer Publishing Company Ltd, London, 1975

Stunkard, A.J., *Obesity*, W.B. Saunders, Philadelphia, 1980

Useful Organizations

Anorexia Nervosa and Bulimia Nervosa

Anorexic Aid
Gravel House, Copthall Corner, Chalfont St Peters, Bucks

Anorexics Anonymous
21 Kitson Road, Barnes, London SW13

Overeaters Anonymous
Pinner: telephone 081-868 4109

The Eating Disorder Association
44/48 Magdalen Street, Norwich

The Elizabeth Gentle Centre
201 Lauderdale Mansions, Lauderdale Road, London W9

Women's Therapy Centre
6 Manor Gardens, London, N7

Maisner Centre for Eating Disorders
PO Box 464, Hove, East Sussex BN3 2BN

Obesity

Weight Watchers Ltd
11 Fairacres, Dedworth Road, Windsor E18

Slimmers Anonymous
The Manor House, Gravesend Road, Shorne, Kent

Index